Early Motherhood in Digital Societies

Early Motherhood in Digital Societies offers a nuanced understanding of what the digital turn has meant for new mothers in an intense and critical period before and after they have a baby, often called the 'perinatal' period.

The book looks at an array of digital communication and content by drawing on an extensive research project involving in-depth qualitative data from interviews with new mothers in the United Kingdom and online case studies. These stories are analysed to investigate the complexity of emotions around birth, the diversity of birth experiences and the myriad ways in which television, the press and social media impede and empower women giving birth. The book asks: what does the use of technology mean in the perinatal context and what implications might it have for maternal well-being? It argues for a balanced and context-sensitive approach to the digital for maternal well-being in the critical perinatal period.

By doing this, the book fills a gap in media studies, addressing itself to gaps within audience analysis, health communication and parenting. It will be essential reading for research and teaching modules in media studies, cultural studies, sociology, health communication and sociology of medicine and health.

Ranjana Das is Reader in Media and Communication, in the Department of Sociology, at the University of Surrey, United Kingdom. Her recent work has focused on parenting, parenthood and technology, with a particular focus on health and well-being. More broadly, she is interested in empirical and conceptual explorations of people's everyday engagement with emerging communication technologies and has researched media audiences and users in numerous projects. Her work has been funded by the Wellcome Trust, the British Academy and the Arts and Humanities Research Council.

Global Gender

The *Global Gender* series provides original research from across the humanities and social sciences, casting light on a range of topics from international authors examining the diverse and shifting issues of gender and sexuality on the world stage. Utilising a range of approaches and interventions, these texts are a lively and accessible resource for both scholars and upper level students from a wide array of fields including Gender and Women's Studies, Sociology, Politics, Communication, Cultural Studies and Literature.

Gender, Heteronormativity and the American Presidency
Aidan Smith

Cultural Representations of Feminicidio at the US-Mexico Border
Nuala Finnegan

Muslim Women's Rights
Tabassum Fahim Ruby

Gender in the 2016 US Presidential Election
Dustin Harp

Latina Outsiders Remaking Latina Identity
Grisel Y. Acosta

Early Motherhood in Digital Societies
Ideals, Anxieties and Ties of the Perinatal
Ranjana Das

https://www.routledge.com/Global-Gender/book-series/RGG

Early Motherhood in Digital Societies

Ideals, Anxieties and Ties of the Perinatal

Ranjana Das

Routledge
Taylor & Francis Group
LONDON AND NEW YORK

First published 2020
by Routledge
2 Park Square, Milton Park, Abingdon, Oxon OX14 4RN

and by Routledge
52 Vanderbilt Avenue, New York, NY 10017

Routledge is an imprint of the Taylor & Francis Group, an informa business

British Library Cataloguing-in-Publication Data
A catalogue record for this book is available from the British Library

Library of Congress Cataloging-in-Publication Data
Names: Das, Ranjana, author.
Title: Early motherhood in digital societies: ideals, anxieties and ties of the perinatal / Ranjana Das.
Description: Milton Park, Abingdon, Oxon; New York: Routledge, 2020. | Includes bibliographical references and index. |
Identifiers: LCCN 2019034550 (print) | LCCN 2019034551 (ebook) | ISBN 9781138052574 (hardback) | ISBN 9781315167725 (ebook) | ISBN 9781351683845 (adobe pdf) | ISBN 9781351683838 (epub) | ISBN 9781351683821 (mobi)
Subjects: LCSH: Mothers—Psychology—History—21st century—Case studies. | Mothers—Social conditions—21st century—Case studies. | Digital communications—Social aspects—Case studies.
Classification: LCC HQ759 .D266 2020 (print) | LCC HQ759 (ebook) | DDC 306.874/3—dc23
LC record available at https://lccn.loc.gov/2019034550
LC ebook record available at https://lccn.loc.gov/2019034551

ISBN: 978-1-138-05257-4 (hbk)
ISBN: 978-1-315-16772-5 (ebk)

Typeset in Sabon
by codeMantra

Contents

Foreword

Mothering experiences were almost entirely absent from public discourse in Britain and North America until around the 1970s, when the Women's Liberation Movement directed long-overdue attention to mothering and maternal labour. Today, however, mothering is impossible to miss. In particular, experiences of early motherhood – the focus of this book – are expressed, depicted, discussed and negotiated publicly across a range of media technologies and platforms. Mothering is intensely mediated.

This book shows what this mediation entails and its consequences during the perinatal stage, that is, before and after birth. Through careful analysis of a range of online representations and texts, including YouTube videos depicting 'hypnobirth', parenting discussion forums and social networking sites and some fascinating interviews with mothers in the U.K., Ranjana Das shows that to understand early motherhood, we must consider its entanglement with media and communication technologies. To make sense of the anxieties, ideals and relationships during that critical perinatal period, we need to situate them within a range of mediated practices: from amateur videos produced by mothers about birthing, to women's postings of birth stories on social networking sites, to mothers seeking advice on breastfeeding from other mothers, in online forums.

But what are the meanings and consequences of the myriad mediated practices documented in this book alongside a growing body of literature on motherhood and digital media? The answers to these questions often fall into the crude binary that has characterised debate on the Internet and the digital from their early days: celebratory and utopian explanations versus moral panic and dystopian accounts.

On the celebratory side of the debate, online technologies and platforms are hailed as empowering and supportive spaces, enabling women to avoid the isolation and sense of helplessness that early motherhood can bring. These spaces are claimed to be liberating, allowing complicated feelings, whose articulation has for long been taboo. On blogs, websites and social networking sites, mothers express not just satisfaction and happiness, but also powerful emotions of frustration, disappointment, dissatisfaction, anxiety, anger and ingratitude. They describe, talk about and critique the unpaid and undervalued onerous work of mothering. Other accounts in the 'utopian' camp emphasise the key contribution of digital parenting social networking sites for critiquing oppressive ideals of motherhood and highlight the role of these sites in destabilising, reframing and politicising the meanings of contemporary motherhood.

On the dystopian side, parenting and especially online mothering forums and sites are depicted as obnoxious, disempowering and sometimes even dangerous places. We are told about the ubiquity and toxicity of mother blaming and mother shaming, and the harsh judgements made of mothers and their parenting practices. The widely used acronym AIBU (standing for 'Am I Being Unreasonable?') on the popular U.K. parenting website, Mumsnet, captures the profound disciplinary role of digital spaces in policing and encouraging the self-policing of mothers' thinking, feelings and behaviour. It is in this context also that the phenomenon of sharenting – posting family snapshots via technology and social media platforms – is often discussed as a key practice through which mothers are scrutinised, regulated and judged.

Early Motherhood in Digital Societies helpfully eschews this binary of euphoric optimism/moral panic around mediated motherhood. Rather, it highlights the multiple, complex and often ambivalent processes, practices and implications of mothers' engagement in and use of digital spaces. We learn about the meaningful camaraderie that emerges across digital spaces and how it is extended to mothers, especially as they reject what they perceive to be oppressive medical advice and technocratic labour cultures. At the same time, Ranjana Das discusses how particular narratives that do not fit the normative 'perinatal ideal', for example, stories of women who had traumatic birthing experiences, are being excluded, censored and silenced. We learn how, in the context of harsh austerity measures and funding cuts that have dramatically reduced the resources for supporting mothers' emotional well-being in the U.K., online spaces offer some sort of lifeline, helping to relieve maternal anxiety in significant ways. At the same time, in the context of neo-liberalism's aggressive push to self-govern and 'self-responsibilise', participating in these online spaces profoundly exacerbates anxiety. Mothers search for the 'perinatal ideal', for instance, the smooth, relaxed, pain-free natural birth, but fail to find it, which results in discord and an agonising sense of personal failure.

The book adds to an important growing field of work that explores the meanings and experiences of mothering in contemporary neoliberal societies. Building on prior work in this area, it highlights the urgency of replacing an individualising and pathologising framework with one that examines and underscores the structural conditions of mothering and how they are shaped inextricably by media practices in everyday life. Thus, rather than calling on mothers to 'fix' or change their feeling, thinking or behaviour, the author makes concrete recommendations about the urgently needed social support structures for mothers, for example, in relation to how the National Health Service's digital strategy could improve maternal well-being.

My hope is that the book will expand our understanding of contemporary mothering, as it becomes increasingly inseparable from the digital sphere and from neo-liberalism and as the notion of biological mothering, on which the book focuses, is being destabilised and complicated in significant ways.

Shani Orgad
London School of Economics and Political Science

Acknowledgements

This book arose out of a significant change, and in many ways, a challenge to my identity with the arrival of little Arjo Blake Hassall-Das. Thank you Arjo for being ever so patient with me and for being a very kind little person.

Many thanks to Adam Hassall for companionship, patience, snack-feeding talents and the funny videos, GIFs and memes with which he keeps me regularly entertained. Particular thanks to Ranjan Das who has made it his mission to be the first buyer of any book I write, and to Sanjukta Das for reading the manuscript through, in its final stages, and to both for being my great cheerleaders in India. And, I am indeed grateful to a furry bundle of chaos, commotion and cuddles called Dizzy!

The work presented in this book has benefited from numerous rounds of peer review and supportive critique. First, my enormous thanks to Shani Orgad for penning the foreword for this book – I am truly grateful! I thank anonymous reviewers at *Social Media and Society, Communication, Culture and Critique, European Journal of Cultural Studies* and *Communication Review*, alongside colleagues at ICA, ECREA and BSA conferences. Various colleagues and friends have read various parts of this work or, on occasion, discussed ideas with me or suggested valuable references. My many thanks in this regard to Elizabeth Anderson, Charlotte Faircloth, Aristea Fotopoulou, Vicki Harman, Chris Hine, Ana Jorge, Sonia Livingstone, Giovanna Mascheroni, Michelle O'Reilly, Nadine Page, Victoria Redclift and Hilde Stephansen. I also thank colleagues at the University of Bergen in Norway – John Magnus Ragnhildson Dahl, Synnove Lindtner – and most importantly Brita Ytre-Arne – my invaluable friend and trustworthy critic, who has many times brought this monograph away from collapsing into the land of self-doubt. I thank colleagues at the Catholic University of Milan, where this work received valuable support and comments, and indeed, colleagues at the University of Surrey, where this work was presented multiple times. Thank you also to Anna Zsubori who provided valuable research assistance at the University of Leicester at an early stage. And, thanks enormously to the British Academy for funding this work.

The Department of Sociology at the University of Surrey has become the warmest home I might have asked for, where colleagues have become friends. I found incredibly useful the two seminars I was invited to give about this work, where I received very valuable feedback from sociologist, criminologist and communications colleagues alike. I particularly thank Vicki Harman and Chris Hine for their detailed reading of the draft manuscript and their invaluable comments and Francesca Menichelli and Giulia Berlusconi for very useful comments on a major empirical chapter from this book. And, I am very grateful to Paul Hodkinson, who has patiently read numerous drafts and has provided wise, kind and thoughtful support by reminding me to 'keep swimming!' through many stop-starts and setbacks.

To the women who let me into their homes and their worlds, thank you more than I can say.

As I was finishing up this monograph, I lost Nayona – my wonderful, sweet, fabulous friend. *Didi*, to your memory, I dedicate this book.

1 Mediated mists of the early days

Autumn-winter, 2015. Bedford, UK.

It is an October afternoon in 2015. I find myself sitting on the steps of our empty house, where, about three days ago, I had gone into labour. My infant son – Arjo – born at the end of 35 hours of labour, is at the hospital, being treated for a presumed infection. He is with his father, who is armed with tiny cups of expressed milk. I have driven out to come home for half an hour, and to get some fresh air and see what the world looked like after the extreme haze of the past couple of days. I have been tutted at by the healthcare staff for coming out for a brief breather.

I sit on the steps and wince in pain. I feel too weak to lodge protests, but I feel profoundly let down that someone around me in the penultimate stages of labour had said, "your contractions are like a cyclist rambling along a residential area. You need to get to motorway speeds in the next hour". I recall being in mind-numbing agony, unable to speak for myself. Little was I to know that, many months later, I would be derided, online this time, by someone else who did not find my birth quite natural enough, for it involved pethidine. My empty house and trembling body, fresh from giving birth, muddle into a blur as I scroll mindlessly through congratulations pouring in on Facebook on the standard new-family picture posted with birth time, birth weight and short sentence of euphoria. The picture shows me smiling, embracing, tired, but delighted. One hundred and forty-five comments. Three hundred and sixty-seven likes and reactions. The picture shows little else.

I login to Skype. My entire family lives in India, and, despite having lived in the U.K. for over a decade, I wish to speak to Indian family members suddenly. I call someone in India, on Skype, and blurt out – *it is all overwhelming – this thing that has just happened.* I am reminded – *but you've got a gorgeous little one now, that must be so wonderful! We are all so thrilled out here!* Elsewhere, congratulatory messages arrive on Facebook, in response to new-family photographs and the usual new-baby announcements with time of birth, and birthweight. I scroll through them for a few minutes, hitting 'like' mechanically on each comment, till my body lets me know that it is time to nurse my infant again and I drive back into the hospital.

Things continue, in a haze. Nights are punctuated with many wakings, online searches for information on everything from cradle cap to nursing positions on YouTube, and periodically lurking on breastfeeding forums, not quite finding the energy to post. Days are filled with checks and queries on my son's growth, his well-being and his weight gain and inquiries from well-meaning relatives about similar things.

Eight weeks later, it is a cold, dark and rainy December day, as I squeeze my car into a narrow alley near a Children's Centre in Bedfordshire. My two-month-old son sleeps peacefully in his car seat as rains lash against the car. Official literature has drilled it into me that I should not be under any pressure to return to a pre-pregnancy body. There is no pressure. I have still not entirely recovered from the birth. Eight weeks on, and my legs still tremble from all the kneeling I did, through the final, extreme, hours of giving birth during the 35 hours of labour. Even driving is a process that involves careful thought, and a great deal of planning about pain-avoiding seated positions. The texture of everyday life has transformed, but I am not unwell enough for a referral to any specialists, I have been told. I look into the rear-view mirror and see myself in a nursing top bought off a Facebook baby and parents' group – in a colour one would normally not find in my wardrobe. I look into my bare eyes, which would usually be done up very deftly with eyeliner.

It is superficial – I chide myself.

It is identity – I answer back.

I hear myself thinking – *everything has changed.*

But there isn't much time to think. I am waiting to meet the Health Visitors, routinely, about my son. Before I go in, I fumble about in the changing bag and bring out the Red Book charting his developmental trajectory and his weight gain. I shine my iPhone torchlight on the page with the centile lines. He is a fine baby, I say to myself, tracking his centile line perfectly. But I cannot quite shake the words I have recently heard from a relative – that he isn't exactly the chubby baby of nappy and baby formula adverts – *is he getting enough milk?* He is. But I again doubt breastfeeding him – *perhaps tracking his centile line isn't enough?* It is, of course, but I do not yet know that these doubts and anxieties would then continue and develop over the next many months.

I quickly open the Mumsnet app on my phone to see if anyone else has responded to my thread, worrying about his weight. Two more people have. One sends a 'hand-hold' and asks me to have a strong, sweet tea. I feel momentarily reassured and confident at this kind gesture (accompanied by the flowers emoji) from an unknown other online. The other respondent reminds me that I am giving him 'the best start in life' and hyperlinks it to evidence that I should continue to do so for the next two years at least. As a social scientist, whose life and work are all about basing convictions in evidence, this piece of hyperlinked, 'authentic' information from the World Health Organization strikes me as very important.[1] But as I stare into the rain on my windscreen, armed with accurate and up-to-date information, I note to myself that I am due to return to work at the end of spring – *I cannot satisfy the WHO guidelines.*

I look around and I see my son smiling and stretching in his sleep. I swipe to the camera of my iPhone and voiceover a quick video of the cute baby and send it off on WhatsApp to my parents in India. It all takes less than a minute. Besotted Indian grandparents (who will not know anything of these anxious moments spent in my car, except a cute, ten-second video of a bonny baby) will soon reply from 3,000 km away. I return to the Mumsnet app, replying to the lady who sent me the WHO link, saying that I will return to work when my son is six months old and I intend to gradually phase out breastfeeding over the first year. Perhaps I sound a tad defensive. There is an immediate reply from the poster – *well, if you must return to work, you have to I suppose.* But, I have two projects I cannot wait to pick up again. The household cannot afford to avail fully of the newly introduced shared parental leave beyond the two months already saved for. Carrying this all in my head, I rush into the Children's Centre. It is very, very busy. One health visitor and two assistants are, with impressive rapidity, weighing babies, plotting them on his record book (the 'Red Book'[2] in the U.K.), passing them on to (largely) mothers to dress them back up – and *next!*

We are next. My son is weighed and plotted. As expected, he is fine. The health visitor is very rushed, and I am conscious of a queue of at least five mums behind me, each bringing in some rain with her, a car seat and at least one displeased baby. The mum standing next to me has already undressed her baby and is pacing, waiting for the scales. I hurriedly dress my son in his many layers, wanting the pacing mum to have the changing mat soon.

The health visitor, trying her very best to keep up with the flow of mums and babies while scribbling on a Red Book, asks me – *and, is mum okay?* I start replying, when she says that I did fine at the six-week postnatal check for mums, so it is all fine.

Is it all fine?

It is time to leave.

Early motherhood: Why the *perinatal*?

This book focuses on early motherhood – which is often referred to as the *perinatal* period – and it considers particularly the pressures and struggles that many mothers encounter in the mist of the early days. The book asks, how do we make sense of the pressures and struggles of the perinatal in a mediated society framework? Why is it important that we do so? My fundamental argument, in response, is that we can only fully conceptualise or investigate these intense months before and after childbirth and the many gendered, responsibilising structural forces at play, and we can only effectively support maternal perinatal well-being in contemporary Western societies if we acknowledge the role of media and communication technologies. Cutting across my findings, I suggest that we understand perinatal ties, anxieties and ideals and their individual and collective dimensions as existing in conditions of mediation, embedded within, shaped by and shaping a range of mediated communicative practices.

'Perinatal' is a term which demands some attention at the outset. It is a largely biomedical term used to refer to the period immediately before and after childbirth, from mid-pregnancy to roughly a year after birth, although a wide variety of definitions prevails. So, indeed, it is predominantly a term one hears within biomedical circles, and yet, I – as a media and communications researcher – use it in this social scientific book. Would *maternal* or something else which sounds less clinical not have done for my purposes in this social scientific work? First, I suggest that, as I develop in greater depth in Chapter 2, the perinatal period – the very useful term for the period immediately before and after birth – encompasses a set of specificities around early motherhood which not only make it sociologically interesting and specific to investigate, but also that these specificities place early motherhood and the maternal under the scrutiny of public and policy microscopes in rapidly successive ways, commensurate with the rapidity of fetal and infant development in the first year, which are not necessarily true for subsequent stages of motherhood. Conception, pregnancy, birth, infertility and neonatal loss in some instances, infant feeding, sleeping, weaning and maternal anxiety and depression regularly feature in public and policy discourse, and mothers find themselves in a position where there is significant rapidity and pace to interfaces with individuals and institutions in the perinatal period. The time frame in question has variable definitions. Some define it as a year before to up to two years after birth (Helfer, 1987), while the period is as small as from a few months before to a week after birth in some definitions (WHO, 1992). For the purposes of this work, which is not a biomedical account but a social scientific one, I keep the period loosely defined as the period before and after birth, leaning closer to Helfer's time frame above. In doing so, I look at a wide variety of experiences of the perinatal, but I pay attention particularly to emotions, mothers' self-reported struggles, their sense of feeling well, experiences of support for perinatal difficulties, interpersonal ties, anxieties and ideals in this period. As the text progresses my focus on mothers experiencing difficulties increases, and I end this book with a focus on a distinct space for the perinatal in the context of the U.K. and its digital health plans, seeking to participate in a broadly biomedical conversation on maternal emotional wellness in the perinatal period from a mediated, sociological perspective.

While this project speaks of *mothers* overall, it is perhaps worthwhile querying the premises behind this. Are mothers a distinct group? Do they and must they perform the tasks of mothering in isolation? What do the terms mothering and motherhood bring that *parenting* does not and vice versa? Some of these questions throw up critical concerns around gendered subjectivities, and others convey normative aspirations in a society seemingly encouraging, but failing to meet the mark, for equal caring responsibilities. I suggest that mothers – as diverse as women's contexts, resources and restraints are – might be considered to be a critical social, cultural and even medical grouping, where attention to the maternal and the myriad structures it functions within and against is indeed justified. As a term, this grouping is employed casually in lay, public discourse, bringing with it a set of norms and expectations which I unpack in this book. But equally, this grouping is mobilised in commercial spaces, medical literature and family, childcare and well-being policies (see Lee et al., 2014, for an excellent critique of policy and institutional discourses in this context). In each of these contexts, women as mothers are framed differently, with varying degrees of responsibilation, as agents or as subjects, as clients or as citizens or as active participants or passive recipients. As scholars from the Centre for Parenting Culture Studies note, policy initiatives appear to place a great emphasis on training mothers, when perhaps mothers may be left to trust their instincts more (Lee et al., 2014). And on the other side, as empirical findings in this book elucidate, maternal instinct might indeed be so celebrated and upheld that exclusive cliques and tribalism might arise, both on and offline, designating the most natural and worthwhile ways in which to mother intensively (Hays, 1998). Public and popular press discourse often valorise and celebrate rhetoric where mothers know best (c.f. Das, 2018), thereby placing enormous value and ideological weight on maternal instinct, not just at the expense of fathers (Brooks & Hodkinson, 2018), and by extension, more egalitarian forms of childcare and responsibility for children, but by feeding into heavily gendered, and pressure-creating logics. Commercial intrusions on social networking sites, such as those inviting women to self-track and self-monitor daily fertility data (c.f. Choe et al., 2014; Lupton, 2016), position women apparently as agents who should be *in control* of their bodies, while commercially exploiting this data and making use of algorithms to direct targeted advertizing to women as clients and consumers, as the shocking incident of Bounty handing on mothers' and infants' data (Hern, 2019) to an array of organisations, draws attention to, as this book is written. This is not just an isolated incident in the context of commercial organisations attempting to profit from pregnancy, birth, labour and the vulnerable first moments of childbirth, nor is it a solitary instance of mothers' and children's data being used for vast commercial gains. These simultaneous and often contrasting articulations of mothers as agents, subjects, clients, citizens, experts and laity, amongst others, make the retention of attention on mothers and the maternal particularly critical.

But motherhood also brings with it a set of often, although not always, early biological responsibilities associated with babies and infants, making the perinatal period stand out particularly. Far from indicating homogeneity with this attention to mothers as a cultural and social grouping, employed in public and policy discourse, and itself bringing with it specificities of the perinatal, I recognise this grouping to be vastly heterogeneous. My focus on mothers and the maternal is intended to be critical of the discourses arising around it, the burdens these discourses place on women, the gaps in provision for mothers' and by extension, families' needs and the uses of communication technologies in this context. Also, I note that while the literature developed for generations on maternity and motherhood is useful, for it incorporates within itself discussions of the history of pregnancy and visual cultures of birthing, I am conscious that using the very term motherhood uncritically in relation to the perinatal alone risks associating motherhood just with the various phases of the prenatal and postnatal periods and excludes the myriad other experiences linked with mothering, including fostering, adoption, fertility treatment, stillbirths, miscarriage and abortion (c.f. Bute, 2009; Bute et al., 2010). So I remain conscious that this book speaks to a small and specific set of experiences of motherhood, by focusing attention on the perinatal, with a particular focus in many instances on mothers' experiences of perinatal difficulties. This book also retains the words *mothering* and *maternal*, for it contends that *parenting* does not grasp the specificities of the (still) gendered norms, responsibilities and expectations of women as mothers in contemporary societies, nor can the physicality and biological aspects of the perinatal be ignored. But while benefiting from the specific focus offered through a focus on mothering and the maternal, I also note that the public and policy emphasis in language on mothers and the maternal simultaneously work to focus attention and expectations systematically on mothers alone. Unless one does indeed use the language of *parenting*, men – in their roles as fathers – are excluded, not only to the detriment of father-child bonding, but also to the detriment of equality in shared childcare, women's return to the workforce and more egalitarian structures in child and infant care, amongst other things (Brooks & Hodkinson, 2019). But nonetheless, as argued above, I hold on to *mothering* and the *maternal*, because for the purposes of this work, it allows recognition and space for women's experiences in the perinatal period and invites critical attention to the discursive and institutional structures which resource or even restrain them.

A mediated framework

> We cannot really isolate the role of media in culture, because the media are firmly anchored into the web of culture, although articulated by individuals in different ways ... The 'audience' is everywhere and nowhere ...
>
> (Bird, 2003, p. 2)

I began this book with a sliver of my own lived experiences of the perinatal period, not (just) because it offered me a small space to let my own self be seen in a monograph where I do not really appear myself. I did so also because this snapshot refers to a range of societal discourses, practices and institutions which will return over and again as this text progresses, and hence this offers me a useful entry point into this work. Just the few snapshots recounted at the start of this chapter, reference maternity and childbirth itself (c.f. De Benedictis, 2017; Tyler & Baraitser, 2013), the physiological and emotional turbulence it often brings, maternal anxiety and its social shaping (c.f. Lee et al., 2014), the shifting support systems and structures in modern Western societies (Coontz, 1997; Litt, 2000) and the role of interpersonal relationships in parenting between mothers and fathers, mothers and other mothers, mothers and internet strangers and mothers and healthcare professionals. It also touches upon diasporas and diasporic communication (c.f. Madianou & Miller, 2013), shared parenting policies, the critical role of fathers not just as supporters of mothers (c.f. Das & Hodkinson, 2019), but also as sole and primary carers in a patchy policy context (c.f. Hodkinson & Brooks, 2018), infant feeding policy, practice and discourse (Faircloth, 2013; Lee, 2008; Wall, 2001), maternal well-being and mental health and the pressures on face-to-face support for mothers and babies (DoH, 2011), to name a few.

But, as Bird's quote above draws attention to, it also refers to these as mediated discourses, mediated practices and mediated institutions, where the proliferation of the latest technologies, through successive waves of the World Wide Web, are shaping practices of parenting, mediating and even shaping public discourse. These interfaces are increasingly being taken up by mothers like myself, as they turn to the Internet in everyday life (Bakardjieva, 2005), not just to engage in laborious practices of what has been termed mummy blogging (Orton-Johnson, 2017; Rogers, 2015), but to engage in what Kleut et al. (2018) term 'small acts of engagement'. These are acts on the go, as support, information and advice are sought and given and anxieties relieved, experienced and shaped in the everyday interstices of maternity and technology. Ley (2007) aptly captures the 'architecture of commitment' afforded on certain online groups drawing upon foregoing conceptualisations of thick trust (Radin, 2006), social capital online (e.g. Haythornthwaite & Wellman, 2002) and techno-socialities (Escobar, 1994). Ley outlines how the very architecture of these groups, including their social and technical design, fosters a kind of commitment and participation that is unique to these digital platforms. A large part of this literature on the social media practices of mothers and parents has focused on framing these as they relate to children's online lives (e.g. Schaan & Melzer, 2015). Mothers' social media habits, including their blogging practices (see Orton-Johnson, 2017), and the sharing of information about their children online (c.f. Chalklen & Anderson, 2017) also sits within this broader context of an interest in mediated parenting (see Blum-Ross & Livingstone, 2017, on 'sharenting'). Distinctively, my focus in this book is more on mother*hood* rather than on mother*ing*, so to speak.

The 'perinatal' period, before and after birth, is mediated by a range of media technologies like all other societal institutions, and increasingly digitally so. The policy context in the U.K., in terms of a series of austerity measures affecting public funding for mothers of very young children on the one hand and the NHS Digital Strategy on the other draws attention both to the emerging gaps in provisions for mothers, and promises, expectations and possibilities around the digital as it is often hailed for its many benefits. In the healthcare sector, health and well-being policy has placed digital technologies at the heart of the agenda, optimistic and charged about their many possibilities (NHS Digital, 2016). And in everyday life, in homes, community groups, through fieldwork also, optimism about information sharing and support finding is evident. Research has evidenced substantially now that women value information and emotional support on well-being related issues in the perinatal period, from accessible, even lay experts online, bypassing or complementing formal sources of information (McKeever & McKeever, 2017; Prescott & Mackie, 2017; Slomian et al., 2017). More generally, women have been shown to be using the internet for health information seeking more than men (Baumann et al., 2017; Myrick & Willoughby, 2017), with good strategies of information seeking online defined as a key health literacy goal (Nutbeam et al., 2017). Online and offline data demonstrated in my own work too that women who had access to the internet valued the sense of agency and initiative that came through self-directed information seeking, often over and above other informal and formal sources of information. Most critically, they found online platforms useful in terms of bypassing waiting periods to be able to access healthcare professionals offline, or even telephone helplines the morning after a difficult night.

Research shows us that offline community support for mothers is declining, given the structure of contemporary societies (Drentea & Moren-Cross, 2005), and in the U.K., NHS-provided offline support – particularly ones which involve women supporting women – is under pressure, and hence also declining (DoH, 2011). But equally, as I go on to elucidate, offline support networks can offer a mixed bag of experiences for women. Media reports note that perinatal mental well-being in general is not considered to be high enough on agendas (BBC, 2018) in terms of public policy, public understanding or acceptance and support in women's professional spheres. In such a context, there has been a proliferation of digital sites of information provision, peer support and mentoring (Cline & Haynes, 2001). The online appears to be an easily accessed realm of information, often even sought as a reflex action, on the go from smartphones. Mapping this on to conversations on digital health divides (c.f. Brodie et al., 2000) and inclusion, one might be inclined to suggest that mothers who are not on these sites or fully participating in them are less equipped to support themselves in issues of well-being in the vulnerable perinatal period. But, is there truth in this claim? More critically, is it the responsibility of struggling mothers, then, to also act as and access the labour of peer support, as structural support for and from the NHS declines? But equally, to consider the intersections of the perinatal and the digital means paying attention to broader representations of the maternal and motherhood in public discourse, looking at responsibilation and individualisation in being ideal mothers and responsible citizens of health and well-being (c.f. Lupton, 2016).

To pick up two instances of groups in the U.K., where such work has laid marvellous foundations which I myself am indebted to, I make particular mention of the CPCS (Centre for Parenting Culture Studies), where scholars have produced ground-breaking work scrutinising institutions, practices and policy discourse around maternity and motherhood drawing out the degree and widespread nature of individualised discourses of responsibilation and mother blame which circulate around us (c.f. Faircloth & Gurtin, 2018; MacVarish & Lee, 2019). The second is the network MAMSIE (Mapping Maternal Subjectivities, Ethics and Identities), which has created a unique, interdisciplinary space for critiquing discourses around motherhood and the maternal, drawing together gender, sexuality, psychology, philosophy and the humanities and social sciences together, more broadly (c.f. Tyler, 2013; Tyler & Baraitser, 2013). I am indebted to both in pondering the role of the digital in the perinatal, as I thought about and wrote this book. I contribute further to these conversations, positioning myself within a framework of mediated communication which invites an understanding of representations, interpretations and communication at the levels of individuals acting in relation to domestic partnerships, in relation to families near and far away and in relation to society, culture, media and communication technologies and the many kinds of private and public institutions involved in all these spheres.

Following Silverstone (1999), Thompson (1995) and Couldry (2004), in this book, I understand mediation to encompass the whole host of communicative practices with media technologies, distinct from either media effects, or simply audience interpretations of texts or even a general comment on media saturation in society. The mediation of the perinatal is necessarily a multipronged process – above and beyond isolated instances of textual representations, snippets of online conversations or focused and specific moments of audience reception of texts. Although this book reflects on some discrete moment from these instances, and instances like these often remain the units of empirical analysis, the process of mediation encompasses all of these and beyond – involving texts, institutions, individuals and societies in multiple lines of interaction. Perinatal mothers, other mothers, partners, midwives, other health care organisations and professionals and relatives and friends as "social actors become progressively dependent on the supply of public meanings and accounts of the world in attempting to make sense of their own" (Silverstone, 2002, p. 762). This beckons attention to how certain stories might be highlighted over others, certain voices silenced, as discourses and narratives of the perinatal develop in society.

Fieldwork

This book draws upon research done for a project which investigated the role of media technologies in the everyday lives of women before, during and after childbirth – and was funded by a grant from the British Academy and the Leverhulme Trust. This work consisted of interviews, in a qualitative research process with 34 mothers, including immigrant women in the U.K. Women were visited usually in their homes and engaged in a semi-structured interview process lasting about an hour, and they came from locations across the middle and south of England, including rural as well as urban locations. This work also consisted of analyses of social media content, such as parenting forums (Das, 2017), videoblogging sites (Das, 2018) and social networking sites (Das, 2017). Women were recruited for fieldwork partly by word of mouth, using social networking sites and forums, and partly with the help of a fieldwork recruitment agency, which used door-to-door visits and questionnaires to find, particularly, mothers from migrant backgrounds, many of whom were not participating on online communities where the initial recruitment took place. Interviews were audio-recorded and transcribed. All material, including material from the online research, was analysed thematically.

Early motherhood in digital societies might appear to construct two monoliths – grouping mothers into a potentially homogenous category and painting a far too broad brush stroke with the term *digital societies*. First, this book is produced out of qualitative research done in the very specific contexts of the U.K. and I read the term digital societies particularly in such a national context. Globally, as the United Nations Millenium Development goals recognise the perinatal period, including but not restricted to a focus on emotional well-being, is recognised to be critical for mothers, infants and families. But in the U.K., with a predominantly state-funded public healthcare system in place (the National Health Service), a series of gaps in perinatal support for mothers have emerged, because face-to-face support for mothers from the NHS is under pressure owing to budget cuts. Health visiting services are struggling in England and conditions are patchier elsewhere in the U.K. (BBC, 2018):

> The birthing centre was full, the actual labour wards were full. So I had to actually give birth on a ward with just the curtain there, which blew ... lots ... but I feel like it was because of that they kind of looked at me and thought, oh this one can just go home and she could just come back later because we're under pressure. And I know they're under pressure. I'm very aware NHS is under pressure and stuff, but that

> always put me off, always made me think well what am I supposed to do. Do I have to now start faking tears before you're going to take me seriously?
>
> Adela

In Adela's case above, the object of a blowing curtain, which would only sometimes protect her from others' gazes, induced fleeting anxiety around privacy. But equally, the curtain – representing a lack of space and overcrowding spoke also of austerity, which had rendered the U.K.'s National Health Service struggling to cope in many maternity wards – and Adela shifted between wider socio-political awareness and her own emotional struggles with lack of privacy as she spoke about the curtain blowing back and forth. Adela's instance here serves as an example of how anxiety in the perinatal is messily intertwined into a variety of structures and relations. The policy context in the U.K., in terms of a series of austerity measures affecting public funding for mothers of very young children on the one hand and the NHS Digital Strategy on the other draws attention both to the emerging gaps in provisions for mothers and promises, expectations and possibilities around the digital as it is often hailed for its many benefits. Indeed, the perinatal period, before and after birth, is mediated by a range of media technologies, like all other societal institutions and increasingly digitally so. But as yet, poor understanding remains, on the brighter and darker sides of the digital mediation of the maternal and the deeply contextual ways in which this needs to be approached. Also, yet, there is not a defined and distinct space for the perinatal in overall digital ambitions in the healthcare sector it seems. Drawing upon conclusions emergent from empirical work with mothers online and offline, this book moves forward from empirical research to produce a set of recommendations for appropriate, constructive and careful uses of technology to support mothers in the critical perinatal period.

But *early motherhood* itself risks constructing a monolith, perhaps. Perinatality was experienced vastly differently by the women I spoke to, and their experiences of the various logics of intensive mothering were highly situated and contextual (see Gillies, 2007, writing on marginalised mothers). Even when one speaks of any particular group of mothers – for instance, when speaking of migrant mothers – one might risk failing to recognise and account for the various intersectional attributes which cut across each other to produce the mediated experiences being spoken of. Conny's anxiety, for example, was affective and sensate to her, in the material spaces of a new flat in Leicestershire, where she was heavily pregnant as a lone parent of two. It was evident as we spoke that a significant part of her chats on Messenger, or her phone calls or texts and even her own online activity was dominated by the subject of her missing slowing fetal movements. She struggled with anxieties around stillbirth, having suffered stillbirth previously – for which she blamed herself, not having spotted the slowing down of movements.

> So I was homeless, pregnant, about 12 weeks pregnant, and then I got the flat, I think, yes, just before I had her, and then she was born at the flat as well. See, even this pregnancy as well, I told them about the movements slowing down. It's changed, like, three times ... that could have been one day where she stopped moving and then, you know, gone.
>
> Conny

Our interview revealed that the conditions which rendered her homeless and partnerless were both heavily classed and gendered, and still fresh and incomprehensibly difficult for her. But the hallways and walls of her new flat continued to remind her of her previous one, from where was evicted and where she lost a relationship and a baby. She repeatedly got herself checked during the new pregnancy, terrified that she would miss slowed movements, for the previous experience had been encoded in her mind as her fault and her doing rather than the classed and gendered circumstances within which had found herself having anything to do with her difficult experience.

In what follows and in the remaining chapters of the book, I attempt to draw out these similarities and differences as I go through individual stories and experiences; but I would like to spend some time, at this point, introducing readers to some of the participants who appear in chapters 5, 6 and 7 of this book. Not everyone who was a part of the project is necessarily a part of this book, and not everyone who is a part of this book receives an equal amount of time and space, for the simple reason that my interviews were very loosely structured around a variety of issues at the intersections of the perinatal and the digital. While non-use and low use are significant in their own rights and appear numerous times, it is often also the case that intriguing accounts of things which unfold when mothers did spend a lot of time online come up, perhaps more often. I will return to these women's stories in greater depth as they appear in the rest of this text, but a broader introduction to them is perhaps useful. I was welcomed into the lives of 34 women, who opened up to me at great length about their perinatal journeys and discussing with me intimate matters, difficulties and struggles, and perceiving me varyingly as distant, academic, stranger or as a fellow mother and sometimes as a fellow migrant mother. While a few of these mothers had what seemed like idyllic journeys through the perinatal and early motherhood, the clear majority spoke of a very wide array of pressures, struggles and attempts to seek support to varying degrees of success.

Some, like Cathy or Leticia, had experienced baby loss, or, like Violetta, were terrified on neonatal loss or, like Layla, had been through infertility, invasive fertility treatments and both had struggled to become mothers. Cathy worked digital technology into her life and her successful pregnancy through a regimen of athletics, fitness and sport, as a means to be in control and on top of everything. Layla shunned much of the world of the online, beyond seeking information. Both, like many others, had a supportive partner and family local to them. Cathy's experiences of researching and attempting to be in control, and believing in strong individual narratives of progress and control over all things perinatal, came up in a variety of cases where mothers felt well and strong – for instance, in Raagini's case. Raagini, a migrant mother, but with many lines of privilege on a variety of different counts, and benefitting also from a supportive family, displayed similar levels of confidence, resilience and familiarity with finding the kind of support she needed online.

Some, like Charmaine, or Elisa and Charlotte, who were much more isolated offline, had entirely divergent experiences when venturing online. Charmaine spoke of the pain and loss she experienced when her high priority natural birth 'failed', and with it, failed a range of social ties which she had carefully built in a natural birthing support group, generating myriad emotional difficulties over and beyond her birth trauma. Elisa and Charlotte, both isolated, found a lifeline on maternity leave and whilst experiencing emotional difficulties, by connecting to online support groups or offline to local mothers they had met online, and it was through such a network that they found not just support for themselves, but great validation in supporting others as they struggled. But many others, who were not isolated offline – for instance, Shamima, a Bangladeshi migrant mother who was tube feeding her sick infants whilst surrounded by an entire house full of relatives who listened to us as we spoke in whispers – felt incredibly surveiled and isolated in the course of their everyday lives, amidst a sea of people in the house. Shamima's lifeline became a cheap calling card to call people back in Bangladesh, while for some others like Moumita, Jaya, Heeya or Hema, not surrounded by a family of relatives, small mobile apps and internet telephony were the extent of connection, both on and offline. Class and privilege cut across migrant mothers' experiences significantly. Privileged migrant mothers such as Kavya and Raagini demonstrated significantly higher levels of engaging with the online and with myriad digital spaces, and both had family support, but for one, Kavya, this support surveiled her nearly as much as it did Shamima.

Some like Elizabeth had their own illnesses to struggle with, for instance, gestational diabetes and resultant complexities, while some like Jemima, Conny or Leiticia had classed, raced and gendered circumstances, which gave them mountains to move whilst they stayed quite significantly offline. Conny's journey through her pregnancies involved eviction, homelessness, abusive partners and an intense urge to monitor every movement and every second of her ongoing pregnancy as we spoke. Jemima spoke of moving homes, haemorrhaging dangerously after her births and coping with multiple young children in her council flat by herself. Leticia's experience of neonatal loss and trauma in Africa, her confused and overwhelmed arrival into the U.K., sorting papers and memories, whilst entirely isolated in a council flat as she progressed through her pregnancy created a degree of difficulty in her circumstances from where seeking support felt very unreachable.

I also encountered wide divergences in degrees of resilience in navigating the world of the online, where cliques, exclusions and competition can be as punishing and as embedded within gendered discourses of intensive mothering (Hays, 1998) as those offline can be – with significant blurring between the two. Those like Gwen or Glenda who felt strong and supported felt able to pick and choose, omit and ignore online rhetoric, as they looked for and settled firmly into spaces which welcomed, in Gwen's case, stories of happy and easy birth, and in Glenda's case, the experiences of large families. Those like Edna or Sofia, who stumbled into groups of anxious and unsupported mothers expected increasingly to be providing each other with peer support, felt rejected and abandoned twice over, once offline and then online. Linda, who came across as one of the most happy and confident participants, was a trained natural birthing instructor herself, and she reiterated over and again to me many of the discourses around ideal births which I speak of in chapters 3 and 4. But none of these accounts can or indeed should be reduced to narratives of individual resilience and strength – far from it. As these accounts above demonstrate, the diversity of contexts, perinatal experiences, backgrounds and the nuanced role of offline support, where simply the presence of a wide network was far from conclusive enough as to the degree of its utility, made for an uneven set of online experiences which I return to in Chapter 7. Whilst I do not expect readers to remember these brief introductions to some of the participants, I attempt, as this book progresses, to tell their stories more broadly as they come up in the course of the text.

While this book does not in the presentation of its findings weave its author into the narrative, I also wished to take some time to write about positionality, in terms of my own journey writing this book. Throughout this project, I have been informed by my own identities as an academic, a parent, a mother, a migrant and a privileged person in cross-cutting ways. The first aspect of these I wished to write about is my own experiences with perinatal well-being. My own perinatal experiences saw me navigate what I can only describe as un-noticed (by both myself and many others) phases of emotional difficulties to do with my own identity, and the myriad ways in which new configurations surrounding motherhood and expectations around it had challenged my sense of self in profound ways. After struggling to find both self and a sense of belonging in my new role, I stumbled upon the array of online spaces for and run by mothers, and moved from lurking to eventually coordinating a few subgroups myself – all pseudonymously.

Despite such pseudonymity, looking back at the end of my participation on such spaces, I know that the value and esteem I found, in supporting others or 'leading' a thread even, provided me a valuable sense of belonging and connection. But equally, I note that much in such spaces is *not* inclusive, and very many practices of motherhood and parenting are often treated with suspicion and contempt. Often misunderstood as wars between individual mothers, the scripts for these, as my research also showed, are rooted in complex social and cultural politics surrounding motherhood, and to blame individual women for competing is to miss the point. Nonetheless, my own experiences of a shattered identity, as Rebecca Asher grasps succinctly in her book (Asher, 2011), coupled with my increasing participation on niche online spaces, where I eventually found some form of belonging, value and esteem amidst myriad unpleasant experiences too, all fed into the kinds of questions which occupied me as I wrote. The shattering of identities, as Asher (2011) notes, links in many ways to the notion of maternal ambivalence (Raphael-Leff, 2010). As I reflected on, in the context of widespread celebrations of 'Mothers' Day' (Das, 2019), uncertainties around the maternal ran through my interviews with most mothers. Some, like Sofia from Algeria, have complicated relationships with mothers elsewhere. Some, like Kavya, are stuck in a loop to be a 'good Indian mother' – learnt within the gentle confines of a warm but not empowering maternal relationship growing up. Some are like Violetta as she wishes to delight in her new baby, but her womb feels like an inhospitable place where a fetus might be 'rejected'. And indeed, such celebrations and many discussions of the maternal often bypass those who have chosen not to be mothers or who cannot be mothers, those who have been mothers once but cannot be mothers again and those who have been mothers but have lost a child. But for many, such ambivalences – ranging from soft uncertainties to powerful emotions that aren't quite 'supposed to be' – go unspoken and unarticulated.

This book is written over a decade into my life as an Indian woman living in the U.K., as a first-generation immigrant with her family of origin all living in India. These were lived experiences I carried into this project from my life in the U.K., but equally, my own past shaped the ways in which I approached this. I was raised in a position of relative privilege, inside an urban metropolis in India, where the perinatal period was both heavily medicalised (in the prevalent urban system of private medical practice) and simultaneously heavily populated by a network of female relatives and elders. The latter is often idealistically and unrealistically positioned as the glorious times of female-led, female-supported networks of birthing and perinatal support, when, to the contrary, my own experiences of watching women go through the perinatal period and the experiences voiced by South Asian mothers in the course of fieldwork were far from solely positive, as many women felt both restrained and surveiled by these vast networks of advice (instructions) and support (monitoring). Growing up, I often found that mothers, under both these frameworks, were positioned largely as needing guidance, whether medical or familial.

Later, my 'coming-of-age', so to speak, in the U.K. was initially in many ways like a breath of fresh air, with the emphasis in NHS discourse on birthing choices and the more informal focus on peer support for natural birthing and breastfeeding. The complexities of these discourses, however, and the lived experiences of intensive mothering cultures (c.f. Hays, 1998) became apparent to me as I progressed through my own journeys with conception, birth and the postnatal. The funding application for the project this book speaks out of (British Academy-Leverhulme Trust funded) was drafted by me shortly before I gave birth myself and its fieldwork done first, during maternity leave and then as the newly returned-to-work mother of a young child. My personal experiences as a communication studies researcher, as a user of the healthcare system in the early years, interactions with countless healthcare professionals and procedures, interactions with mothers and my engagement with online forums spoke unavoidably at two levels to the intellectual priorities that emerged during the process of research. At one level, my participants engaged with me very often not just as a researcher who had walked into their living rooms with a notepad and a voice recorder, but also, as I realised very early on, as a mother of a very young child. This meant that transcripts often showed instances where responses would assume my familiarity with problems, challenges and potential solutions.

At another level, as a migrant South Asian woman myself, my positionality in interviews with migrant mothers was particularly critical. Some mothers were delighted to be able to speak in their (our) native languages, while to some, resident in the U.K. for generations, this was insignificant. Some welcomed me as someone speaking their language, as a fellow mother, to whom home-cooked pickles and sweets could be offered as refreshments. My field notes from these interviews reveal now that I left these encounters feeling warm and connected to my work and life in the U.K. Others interpreted me as the expert analyst, the professional woman, perhaps even an expert with solutions to offer rather than someone who could be welcomed informally. It was critical here to note that, especially when interviewing mothers who felt isolated, both socioculturally and linguistically, I had to work to maintain my distinctions between my role (that of a researcher, who would not be able to provide direct solutions or help of any kind) and that of a professional, for instance, whose task it is to provide support.

These reflections on positionality ultimately stay outside the way I compose the rest of this book – the writing of which, in many ways, has often brought a variety of issues very close home for its author. To embrace this fully and entirely would possibly have been a brave choice. A different text might have resulted had I followed Elliott's honest account of the weaving in of her own identity, networks and reflections into her project with mothers (2011), drawing upon Baraitser's (2009) use of her own maternal experience to inform her research. Elliott's exposition of the researcher as instrument is meaningful here: "Data are produced through what the she is able to hear, what she thinks to ask, what she avoids, pursues, remembers and forgets, and importantly, through what she feels" (p. 1). But, doubtless, my own interest in the subject has emerged out of the earliest two decades of my life spent in an Asian metropolis, surrounded one might argue by what Kitzinger called the 'technocratic cultures of birth', with my own childbearing adulthood spent in Britain decades after the achievements of the natural birthing movement had been established and much of these embraced into the NHS system of maternity care. This provided a reflexive opportunity to witness and experience both birthing cultures as an insider and, for the latter, also as a migrant mother. My introduction to birthing and parenting classes, the literature, the information leaflets, the friendly conversations with fellow mothers pre- and post-birth and my participation on online forums and groups all created the backdrop against which this project emerged. My own experiences as a birthing mother, who sought and valued privacy in birthing, and then as an academic mother navigating evidence-based information and advice online while coping with the affective and emotional dimensions of online relationships, advice-giving and support were all elements I brought into this project.

A synopsis of this book

In this book, I draw upon findings from qualitative research, trying to grasp the role of media technologies, particularly digital technologies, and environments in the context of perinatality. Across my empirical chapters, I argue that we make sense of perinatal ties, anxieties and ideals in its individual and collective nuances as embedded within, shaped by and shaping a range of mediated communicative practices. As I have alluded to previously, I speak often of difficulties, struggles and a range of burdensome mediated social structures shaping the experiences of perinatality in the U.K. and potentially in a variety of other societies. I also speak, on occasion, of supportive ties, bonds and solidarity and areas where dominant discourses are resisted and genuine solidarity results. But all inclusions can be exclusive, and the morally heavy nature of much about the perinatal means that no sites of resistance can be approached through a single lens.

My approach to exploring the mediated conditions in digital societies, in which perinatal experiences are born, centres on the notion of the *perinatal ideal* which derives from and is maintained by the logic of intensive motherhood (Hays, 1998). I discuss this notion in Chapter 2. Here, I conceptualise the perinatal ideal as inherently mediated, where life in digital societies is seeing significant transformations in structures of representations, connections and intrusions in relation to the perinatal. I conceive of the perinatal ideal as an individualising, responsibilising and morally weighted set of conditions which traverses a multitude of objects and spaces in the perinatal years. Located firmly within the intensive motherhood ideology (Hays, 1998), it derives its specificity from the biological and practical conditions and logics of the perinatal period itself.

I make use of the frameworks mobilised in Chapter 2, as I present the rest of the book. In various chapters of this book, I consider the role of moralising discourses which create inclusions for some and exclusions for others, under conditions where the perinatal mother must remain tied to the infant as an indicator of 'good' mothering. Chapter 3 does this by looking at the notion of the perinatal ideal through an illustrative analysis of the perinatal ideal as it operates in amateur YouTube videos portraying a specific style of natural births called hypnobirths, which make use of relaxation and hypnosis techniques during labour and birthing and offer an alternative to birthing in interventionist, obstetrics-led settings. Moving forward from the visible advantages of relaxation and hypnosis-related birthing support within the context of the natural birthing movement[3] to restore women's agency in birthing, resisting and rejecting hyper-medicalised technocratic cultures of births, this chapter suggests that these home-made, amateur hypnobirthing videos need to be viewed against the feminist critique of the intensive motherhood discourse, which sees the videos producing the birthing mother as an individualised, self-regulating and highly invested neo-liberal subject, transcending pain in a mythic journey of blissful birthing.

Such discourses of individualisation which responsibilise mothers over and again return in Chapter 4, which looks at the articulation of the perinatal ideal in the specific contexts of childbirth across a set of two online platforms – discussion forums and social networking sites, reading these against discussions about the self-managing, intensive mother who is responsible for making the very best decisions for her child. I consider the work done here to silence and shut down as 'horror stories', experiences which do not fit into narratives of 'good' birthing. Online discussions of birthing display the juxtaposition of two value-laden narratives, deeply linked to each other at times, where inclusiveness produces exclusiveness, so to speak. The one side emphasises the necessity and superiority of a drug-free vaginal birth and sits within the feminist rebuttal of obstetric domination of birthing and is an empowering discourse. The other seems to seek to silence those whose births did not fit within this model and presents them with the task of muting the 'horror-story' narrative. I argue in this chapter that the morally intense nature of some online environments within broader, gendered structures of perinatality necessitate caution in place of assuming that all peer support spaces online are uniform or uniformly useful.

The discursive pressures of the perinatal ideal return again in chapters 5 and 6. Chapter 6 looks at the mediation of maternal anxiety, something which lies at the heart of concerns around maternal depression in the perinatal year. Maternal anxiety, particularly in the 'perinatal' period before and after childbirth, has long interested professionals, the popular press and public discourse, usually as an individualised, clinical condition, which is linked via discourses of inferred blame to its impacts on the fetus/infant. I problematise this and argue that in contemporary digital societies, we must study perinatal anxiety in a mediated, sociological framework, shifting or at least complementing the locus of attention and support from individual mothers to mediated structures. I present my findings in three strands. First, I speak of the 'red herring of infant well-being', where I demonstrate how, in digital societies, perinatal anxiety often manifests, finds reassurance and is produced and maintained in the guise of highly specific infant well-being related issues, but is essentially rooted in ideals and ideologies surrounding mother blame. Second, I focus on 'discourses of support as discourses of responsibilisation' – where I consider supportive resources within the world of online peer-to-peer support, which appear to ease, but sometimes actually maintain the conditions for anxiety by responsibilising mothers. I suggest we step away from individualised, pathologised, blame discourses of anxiety by focusing attention on the infrastructures of anxiety in contemporary mediated societies.

Throughout the book I consider also the empowering and positive aspects of perinatal mothers' engagement with the digital. Online spaces offer valuable information and support for struggling mothers and many of these spaces open up genuine online and offline avenues for perinatal mothers for connection, resistance and mutual support. Chapter 4 findings reveal, for instance, powerful sites of agency and resistance against dominant, often hyper-medicalised discourses, where online discussions offer a cathartic, empowering and questioning space as women prepare for and make sense of childbirth. But I note also that counter discourses are complex, many inclusions produce exclusions and vice versa. I observe that digitally mediated connections might positively complement rework or reshape existing offline support networks. Such findings come up, for instance, in Chapter 5, where I discuss interpersonal ties in the perinatal period and present findings on how offline networks and relationships are often mediated through online means and connections.

The book traces discourses around the perinatal through mothers' interpersonal connections, both on and offline, with doubtless blurring between the two. Chapter 5 foregrounds these connections and considers the ways in which discourses revolving around the notion of the perinatal ideal mediate social ties. In general, I find that the role of offline support networks is complex and should not always be assumed to be supportive, as a range of exclusionary, pressure-creating and moralising discourses might be part of the very support networks women engage with both online and offline. I present findings in Chapter 5 on the moral weight of motherhood in contemporary societies, rendered particularly visible in the perinatal period, which complicates a central boundary in the study of online interpersonal relationships between information and communication. I also note the relative significance, in emotional terms, of temporally contained social ties in digitally mediated perinatal connections. None of these can be approached in solely positive/emancipatory or negative/restrictive terms, but rather showcase the perinatal as a site of meaningful, mediated interpersonal connections. Throughout the book I note that interpersonal ties in the perinatal are shaped by online experiences and short-lived online ties are often affectively significant.

Chapter 7 presents my overall claims and findings from the empirical work this book presents. In particular I draw out a set of key conclusions as I think through the implications of digital technology for perinatality, focusing first on unevenness in contexts of access and use of the digital, a case for optimism in thinking about perinatality and the digital and a case for caution. I note that intersectional experiences within easy-to-form groupings of perinatal mothers must remind us not to reduce digital access, literacies and practices to individual narratives of success or failure. Many mothers are not online, many who are online appearing to seek information only and not support, and telephony continues to be significant. Balancing these various factors, overall, my findings lead me to elucidate why the digital come to matter for perinatality and how this is far more nuanced and far less straightforward than might be expected. I suggest that the transformations we live through in digital societies mean that perinatality itself is seeing changes in representations, connections and intrusions, all of which have significant shaping roles to play in mothers' experiences of the perinatal. I conclude this book by reading my findings in the context of gaps in care in terms of perinatal well-being in the U.K. I argue that recent austerity measures and funding cuts have resulted in gaps in provision, owing to which healthcare professionals, who are already focused on both mothers and infants or very young children (as opposed to mothers alone), are stretched, and provisions for mothers' emotional well-being but also wider forms of support around the myriad difficulties and challenges in the perinatal period are equally stretched. Here, in making recommendations, my argument is that digital perinatal or maternal well-being needs neither the reinvention of wheels nor great aspirations around the digital, but that balancing optimism and cautious perspectives might allow us to make a clear and strong case for the role of digital interfaces in filling critical, emerging gaps in perinatal support and well-being, at least in the U.K.

This book pays attention to mediated practices and discourses within the perinatal period in women's lives in the U.K. This means that in keeping with developments in media and communication studies, the question of interest to me is not the effects of individual texts or representations as such, or audience understandings of specific textual discourses or mothers' use of any particular platforms alone – although these must appear, and indeed they do, as units of empirical exploration in this text. Rather, my focus is on mediation – the broadest range of practices which are "oriented towards media and the role of media in ordering other practices in the social world" (Couldry, 2004, p. 115) – reading media here as 'digital' primarily for the purposes of this work. Using research done in a Western industrialised society – the specific context of the U.K. – I aim to make sense of early motherhood in digital societies by broadening out the focus from texts, audiences and institutions to the wider variety of mediated, communicative practices, only a few of which I can pay attention to in this work.

Notes

1 The frequent reference in many similar communities to WHO guidance on breastfeeding often ignores the fact that a large part of breastfeeding guidance relates to the notion of 'generalised' risk of formula feeding, when in reality much of these risks are associated with regions experiencing lack of access to clean water and hygienic conditions for the safe preparation of infant formula (see also Wolf, 2011).

2 As I finish this monograph, plans have been announced for the Red Book to go digital (BBC, 2018, see here www.bbc.co.uk/news/health-46701196, link accessed last on 29.04.2019). This is intended to make life simpler for parents and healthcare providers, although it remains to be seen what happens in terms of the digitalisation of the significant amount of data in question. For my own experiences above, the materiality of the Red Book and the physical plotting of weight gain on the centile lines were significant in contributing to the affective experiences at Health Visitor clinics.

3 Following Mack (2016), it is important to note that "the use of the term natural to describe home birth or unmedicated vaginal birth is highly contested. The term, some have argued, denotes that other forms of birth are unnatural, wrong, or inherently problematic" (p. 64).

2 The perinatal ideal

In this chapter, I construct a framework, exploring a network of ideas following broadly two central notions in sociology and communication studies. I bring together a conceptualisation of the perinatal ideal – a mediated, responsibilising, individualising set of conditions, an ideology which, I suggest, produces an infrastructure for perinatality which burdens women in their roles as new mothers in cross-cutting ways. I construct part of my framework for the perinatal ideal from within feminist sociology, weaving together a range of concepts around the maternal, pivoting broadly around the decades of scholarship on intensive mothering (Hays, 1998). I position this alongside the central idea of mediation (Silverstone, 1999; Thompson, 1995) from communication studies, which has established an array of concepts with which to make sense of the intertwining of the social and the digital. Bringing the two together, the intention is to embed decades of sociological research with the perinatal into decades of work on mediation and to construct a relationship of mutuality.

The intensive perinatal

Much of what follows in this section owes a debt to the theorisation of intensive mothering – a term which was coined in 1998 by Sharon Hays to represent a group of widely held beliefs about the necessity of mothers investing vast amounts of emotional labour and energy into raising their children, which went above and beyond the perhaps obvious strength of emotions that might usually exist between mother and child (Arendell, 2000; Miller, 2007). Intensive mothering fits perfectly into heavily gendered, neo-liberal visions of individual responsibility and self-management, where overworked mothers must remain tied to the priceless child. It is theorised to tease out how individual parenting practices both feed into and from this discourse, as the discourse is increasingly also taken up and promoted at institutional levels (see Harman et al., 2019). Historically this has been a highly raced and classed discourse, driven strongly by white, middle-class values, which has later been critiqued in analyses of mothering in young, low-income communities (e.g. Romagnoli & Wall, 2012) and in black communities (Elliott et al., 2015; Hamilton, 2017). As several scholars point out (Bruer, 1999; Harris, 1998; Nadesan, 2002), this discourse has been mobilised at various private and public institutional levels placing a strong imperative in the hands of mothers to invest high amounts of physical and emotional energy into specific activities and practices with children, without which they might themselves be putting their children's interests last or undertaking enormous risks.

As is evident from the scholarship on parenthood and risk (Gong, 2016; Lupton, 1999; Petersen, 1997), this positions two kinds of risk. The first positions a heightened sense of risk in all aspects of child-rearing simply by establishing the one, right, good way of parenting/mothering. The second aspect of risk (see also Lupton, 1999, for an excellent discussion) here involves groups who are outside of what is a predominantly middle-class discourse (see Fox, 2009; Wall, 2010), and therefore positioned as at risk (see Lee et al., 2010; also Gillies, 2007; Furedi, 2008). This includes young mothers who are often the subject of reality television shows (see Macvarish, 2010), mothers from lower-income communities or from non-White backgrounds, when many of the choices and practices encouraged and held in high regard within the intensive mothering discourse may not be available or accessible to certain groups. Chae (2015), in an analysis of Korean mothers, reveals the uptake of the intensive mothering discourse primarily within middle-class women, who also drew from celebrity mothers in terms of inspiration. It is crucial to note here though that findings from mothering, return to work and childcare practices in Chile (Murray, 2014) reveal lower-income groups embracing the intensive mothering ideology more so than middle-class mothers. As Murray notes, this is a "contrast with the assumption of a dominant parenting ideology of the privileged middle class (Hays, 1996) – both local and global – operating as the starting point for evaluating the rest" (p. 1173). Butler's engaging (2010) analyses of mothering practices and ideology in British Columbia reveals how state regulatory literature subtly works in intensive mothering and frames parenting practices in general as deeply individual responsibilities within their 'Investing in Children' framework, marking a clear shift from a previous approach to parenting which followed a 'family responsibility' framework (see also Furedi, 2006a, on 'cotton wool' kids).

This discourse sits within the broadly neo-liberal contexts of its shaping and development, and in the specific context of the U.K. with a state health service – the NHS. This development has particular socio-political significance in relation particularly to the recession of state-funded perinatal support for mothers on the ground. Neo-liberalism (Giroux, 2008) and its focus on viewing societies, publics and communities primarily as markets and consumers works by the retreat of the state towards becoming a small state (c.f. Brown, 2015; Larner, 2000; Vesnic-Alujevic et al., 2018) and places responsibilities of self-management and discipline on individuals, which in this case relates to parents, but mothers at large.

As Rose elucidates clearly, as the state retreats, relationships between state and individual (as individuals and communities) begin to shift the locus of responsibility on to individuals presumed largely to be self-disciplining, self-managing consumers (Rose, 1999). In terms of maternity and motherhood, the critical role this discourse plays, as its seeps out into the everyday division of labour at home, childcare responsibilities and sundry household roles, is notable, as Coltrane (2010) points out. Much of this is poignantly captured by Shani Orgad in her book *Heading Home* (2019), as she discusses the 'choices' made by women who give up careers to stay at home and the *lack* of choice inherent in the very word 'choice'.

But these outcomes, emergent from the confluence of as well as feeding into a whole range of discourses, of course, are far from benign. Evidence exists from within psychology that discourses of idealised mothering and motherhood have a role to play in the emotional well-being of mothers (Hewitt & Flett, 1991; Rizzo et al., 2013; Stoeber & Otto, 2006). The takeaway from these studies has usually been that women should not be subscribing to perfectionist ideals about mothering, placing responsibility on women for the uptake of such ideals rather than investigating the ways in which these ideals are transmitted and maintained within society. Critical-cultural, feminist and broadly sociological interventions in the area provide a way out of this individualised placing of responsibility for women's emotional health on themselves, by offering critiques of the mediated transmission and reproduction of these discourses.

The clearest area where mothers' emotional health finds public and institutional recognition is in the realm of perinatal mental health, in particular postnatal mental health. While studies exist in obstetrics trying to find linkages between mode of birth and postnatal emotional health, what escapes is an evaluation of the relationships between the ideals and expectations with which women walk into the perinatal period, itself replete with individualised and hyperconscious awareness of their own prenatal roles and preparations (supported also by institutions), and their emotions post-birth or their experiences of how the perinatal goes for them in reality. Ellie Lee's (2008) and Charlotte Faircloth's (2013) findings on infant feeding practices do precisely this task of complicating a terrain which involves women's bodies so centrally. The focus, as later chapters elucidate, should perhaps be on the simultaneity of recognising women's voice and agency in the face of a medicalised, technocratic discourse, when reflecting both in micro and macro terms on the ideals, expectations, disappointment and blame in the earliest days of the mothering experience, where even before giving birth, standards have been set that are to be aspired for, to be the proper, good mother. This duality, which I discuss as almost two sides of a coin, might be conceptualised, however, as discussions of empowering discourses about knowing one's body and baby versus neo-liberal discourses around attached, involved, invested and heightened forms of care, which frames multiple mediated facets of the perinatal today.

Conceptualising the social constructions of expectations, anticipations and pressures within which contemporary motherhood in the U.K. operates while drawing upon literature around intensive mothering, we must note also that the phenomena behind these discourses and practices of course predate their labelling (see, for instance, Smith-Rosenberg and Rosenberg's historical account on the 'female animal' in 19th-century America). But recent historical shifts in the division of domestic labour, the perception and mediation of mothers' bodies and the relationships between birthing, pregnancy and consumer culture have undergone massive changes in relation to other political, economic and cultural logics, and some of these discourses have become more visible, pronounced and mediated over the recent past (c.f. Bochantin et al., 2010; Douglas & Michaels, 2005; O'Brien Hallstein, 2011; Moravec, 2011; O'Donohoe et al., 2013 Tyler, 2009). This includes work by Joan Wolf (2011), for instance, as she speaks of the relationships between various components of perinatality and notions of responsibilisation and perceptions of risk in neo-liberal societies, particularly as they lead to regulatory rhetoric. I also draw attention to Douglas and Michaels (2005) on 'the new momism', work by O'Brien Hallstein (2011) on 'bikini-ready moms' and feminist scholarship in Britain by McRobbie (2013), Littler, (2013, 2019) and Tyler (2009) on the political-economic and cultural contexts, within which maternal subjectivities are produced and maintained and mother blame and guilt rationalised. Such an individualised, idealised maternal subjectivity privileged within the intensive motherhood discourse (Hays, 1998) draws attention to maternal labour as a coherent set of tasks and functions (Ruddick, 1989) and focuses on the unconscious intersubjective dynamics involved in motherhood (Hollway, 2001). This links to conceptualisations of 'good' mothering and 'bad' mothering, which in turn link to 'deviancy' debates on good and bad parenting as strongly classed discourses of neo-liberalism (Jensen, 2012). Douglas and Michaels (2005) speak precisely of this in the American context, as they define new momism as "a set of ideals, norms, and practices most frequently and powerfully represented in the media, that seem on the surface to celebrate motherhood, but which in reality promulgate standards of perfection that are beyond your reach" (p. 5). These unattainable ideals feed into the systems that keep placing mothers with the greater responsibility or even burden of primary care. Discourses about 'competitive mothers' are illuminating in this context, as they unhelpfully place a focus on individual women rather than calling attention to structure, but also in a world where fetus and infant is a celebrity and considered priceless, the mother is tied to that individualised end product. These then feed into on and offline discussions becoming heavily moralised and all issues of the perinatal becoming affectively impactful.

Of enormous value here are decades of feminist scholarship on maternal subjectivity, including the abjection of maternal subjects in feminist theory, the disappearance and erasure of the maternal to make way for the fetal celebrity (Tyler, 2013) and the subsequent rise of the hyper-mediated new maternal visibility and its own cultural politics of positioning the neo-liberal maternal self. Kristeva's theorisation of primary narcissism, which draws our attention to the seemingly unproblematic unity of mother and child, or Arendt's work on natality link straight on to Tyler and Baraithser's work on the visual cultures of pregnancy and maternity and on feminist media, on cultural studies work by Gill and McRobbie on the neo-liberal maternal self and on Hays' work on theorisations of intensive motherhood. Each beckons attention in their own ways to mothers as self-disciplining subjects (Gill, 2007; McRobbie, 2009), erecting problematic ideals of good and bad mothering, built around narratives of sacrifice where the perinatal is the site of multiple 'body projects' (Tyler & Baraitser, 2013). Tyler and Baraitser (2013) note: "if pregnancy was previously imagined as a passive, abject and ordinary physical state to be stoically borne in private, today pregnancy is a disciplinary 'body project' which women are instructed to covet and enjoy" (p. 23). Jensen's critique of the genderless word 'parenting' is particularly valuable to conceptualise the perinatal, because deleting the physical realities of the gendered nature of the bulk of parenting that falls on the mother – with pregnancy, birth and early infancy as the space where this becomes biologically clearest – is problematic in its own ways.

Audiovisual imagery made possible insights into fetal development, which have been critiqued for their erasure of a focus on maternal development apart from her identity as a vessel for the fetus (Stabile, 1992), generating what Parker (2009) calls the 'maternal ideal', premised upon the hailing of an emotional inability/unwillingness of the mother to ever separate from her baby. Tyler (2013) terms this the fetal celebrity, which renders mother to nothing but vessel. It relates to the appeal of trackable, traceable, fetal and infantile development, which as (Parker, 2009) succinctly argues, leaves stranded any attention to maternal well-being except in relation to that of the infant. Parker works through how this links to the notion of change and how change in the perinatal is conceptualised largely in terms of the child, not the mother. This last, in particular, finds specific meaning and relevance in Chapter 6, where I look at the cultural coding of perinatal anxiety against the backdrop of broader conversations on postnatal depression in women. Throughout the empirical chapters, I present Parker's term (2009) the 'maternal ideal' – an emotional inability to ever separate from her baby – emerges in myriad forms and underlies the mediated logic of the perinatal ideal I speak of in this book. So, fetus and infant gain identity and attention, but mother disappears, it seems.

Shifting geographies and overlapping cultures of birthing, perinatality and migration (Gedalof, 2009) come into play repeatedly in migrant mothers', particularly first-generation migrant mothers, accounts of the perinatal and its difficulties. As I spoke to them, myself as a migrant mother, what came across often was culturally coded accounts of maternity and mothering in our conversations, where home and away blurred and blended, the performance of motherhood in the sleep-deprived early years, often speaking simultaneously to parallel cultures, sometimes similar and sometimes different, yet almost always resourcing anxiety through a range of in/formal discourses. Leticia, who appears later in this book, exemplifies a few of the complexities and overlaps in negotiating the perinatal when being part of two contexts at least, and yet potentially not quite rooted anywhere. She spoke at length about her experiences of neonatal loss whilst in Africa and then her subsequent maternity in the U.K.:

> There's so much difference between emotional support in Africa and emotional support in the UK. Because girls (in Africa) are expected to be strong ... Come on, you just had a baby; get on with it, you've ... I've had ten.
>
> Leticia

Leticia is a new mother, who has arrived in the U.K. from Africa. She recounted to me the harrowing experience of giving birth in a crowded hospital and being told that her baby had died, but then, never seeing any 'proof' of the baby's death, let alone seeing her baby at all. As a very young mother, with little practical resources to support her, she then spent a vast amount of time looking for her baby in the hospital. She recounted postnatal memories of living in a communal compound, with her mother around, who in her attempts to make Leticia be *strong*, erased all references to her missing baby.

> She wanted to make me strong you know as a mother. As a woman. She never spoke to me about the dead baby, nothing. She would come and find me crying because we lived in the same compound. She would find me crying; she would never even care why I'm crying, even ask me or nothing. And the stuff that I had bought for baby, when she was coming to get me from hospital she took everything away from me.
>
> Leticia

For her next birth, this time in the U.K., the corridors of the London hospital where she was due to give birth made Leticia repeatedly subsumed by anxieties around baby loss, both in terms of neonatal death as well as in terms of very physically losing the infant from her sight. But things then went well, and she experienced the U.K. to be more emotionally supportive as she battled anxieties around baby loss rooted in her harrowing trauma. But she still remembered on very many occasions the necessity to 'be strong' no matter what – her own, learnt, referential framework which erected for her, quite like the other mothers in this section, a yardstick against which a mother must perform perinatality to perfection, even when coping with significant trauma.

Feminist migration scholarship on reproduction and issues of collective social identity raised by migration and diasporas in relation to the home, mothering and caring is of note in the context of this work. Ryan's work (2007) on mothers juggling and juxtaposing local and transnational networks, Salih's (2003) attention to the emotional labour inherent in such juggling and maintenance work and Gedalof's (2009) querying and deconstruction of the twin and seemingly stable notions of 'here' and 'there', of 'local' and 'global' are key here. As Gedalof (2009) poignantly argues:

> The question is not only how migrant mothers are constrained by pre-existing structures in their agency, but also, how can we understand both structures and agents of belonging as messy and dynamic entanglements of constraint and enablement, being and becoming, movement and inhabitance.
>
> (p. 88)

This shifts the focus away from manufacturing home and elsewhere as stable sites, with mothering going on in-between to produce a third stable site, and moves towards locating the "dynamism within the work of reproduction and motherhood itself" (Gedalof, 2009, p. 88).

As Lee's analysis of infant feeding and maternal identity (2008) reveals, both giving birth and breastfeeding are complex issues in terms of representations of the maternal in public and policy discourse. Both share two facets which are rooted strongly in biological facts. A medically unintervened vaginal birth, where the woman has had the opportunity to make her own informed decisions, progress at her own pace through labour and be supported by the medical community as and when required, is, as many would argue, a better outcome than one where women's voices are muted by obstetricians wearing white coats, demanding women lie on their backs and 'get on with it'. And yet, this positions birth almost as a binary – where there can be nothing in between what is deemed to be a fully, natural, unassisted birth and a birth where women's voices are muted by obstetricians. Likewise, human milk, tailor-made for human babies, possessing maternal antibodies, many argue, cannot be replicated fully by formula milk. And yet, infant feeding is a far more complex matter than simply what goes inside the infant's body, as it involves wider moralising discourses (c.f. Lee, 2008) and the mother's own well-being. Then, both childbirth and breastfeeding have been at the heart of capitalism – private medical practice and the nexus of privately paid gynaecologists in many Asian cities, for example, ensure most births are Caesarean sections, and the politics of formula circulation, supply and promotion are staggering. But many of these debates need repositioning and reworking in other contexts, for instance, where healthcare is largely state-provided and where water and hygiene conditions make for very different contexts of formula feeding than in those countries where the availability of clean water is a significant issue.

In relation to birthing, in the U.K., we saw a critical, feminist intervention that sought to restore women's voices in the labour room, for justifiable reasons. As Sheila Kitzinger (2012a) pointed out, the return of attention and energy to women's agency in birthing was a rebuttal of the technocratic culture of medicalised birth. Kitzinger led what was to become a movement from individuals and institutions in some cases, although not all, to recognise that in the "technocratic system, birth usually takes place in an alien environment among strangers, with routine use of invasive procedures that are promoted by multinational drug and equipment companies" (2012a, p. 301). This feminist critique of obstetrics-led birthing represented a powerful rejection of masculine structures of dominance over women's bodies, where women's choice and agency in birthing were erased (Oakley, 1984; see also Takeshita, 2017; Winderman, 2016).

Contemporary iterations of the natural birthing movement have, however, been critiqued also from feminist frameworks (Brubaker & Dillaway, 2009; Mack, 2016) about establishing a normative and ultimately controlling narrative of the way women must carry pregnancies, birth and mother, extending from pre-pregnancy preparations, birthing through to infant feeding and sleeping. Mack's poignant analysis (2016) of home-birth videos revealed these to be "self-made narratives that reinforce dominant discourses of masochistic motherhood in a neoliberalist context that conditions mothers to self-renounce, self-deny, and sacrifice in order to be 'good' citizens" (p. 47; see also Cripe's, 2017, autobiographical account on the stigmas of C-section births). These findings are consistent with the discussion on 'sacredness' in birthing in Klassen's (2001) analysis of births outside of medical settings, Chadwick and Foster's (2013) account of the ideal of natural childbirth and the good mother imperative and with Wall's (2001) analysis of social documentation on breastfeeding revealing "a neoliberal preoccupation with individual responsibility" (p. 1). While the vast majority of these practices originated as a legitimate, feminist, critical response to medicalised systems which may work to remove women's choice, the new, 21st-century, hyper-mediated discourse of an idealised perinatal generates its counterpart of the failed ideal. This comes up also in Malacrida and Boulton's findings (2012) in interviews with mothers and childless women, which revealed selflessness as a key attribute of women's perceptions of motherhood, ascribing the embracing and transcending of pain as an essential criterion for that to happen, and by default, writing in a narrative of failure into perinatal processes and events which deviate from the established ideal. The relationships between motherhood, selflessness and sacrifice within the intensive motherhood discourse (Hays, 1996) have been critiqued within feminist frameworks across the spectrum, from pregnancy to child raising. Intensive mothering discourses and their production and maintenance of good and bad mothering not only sustains deeply gendered norms of parenting, but privilege certain styles of mothering over others by creating narratives of good and bad, which become referential frameworks for how mothers interpret their choices and lives (Hays, 1996; Miller, 2007).

At its broadest level, like intensive mothering, I think of the perinatal ideal as an ideology which places a great burden on women as they go through early motherhood, working through deeply gendered logics, and in ways which are produced, maintained, repeatedly re-enacted and circulated and potentially, indeed, resisted, through media and communication technologies. It derives its niche, I suggest, from the now heavily moralised, biological specificities of perinatal fetal and infant development (c.f. Faircloth, 2013; Lee, 2008), thus deriving such a specificity from the precise conditions of the perinatal, which are closely linked but barely restricted to the pace of biological change in the period. At one level, of course, the specificities I mention in terms of conditions of the perinatal derive from the unique rapidity of infant development which occurs in the first year post-birth, and the intense, acute and heightened interfaces with policy and practice in infant well-being and healthcare, with ever-increasing technological advancement that parents, but particularly mothers, go through. Bion (1965), decades ago, called pregnancy a *catastrophic change* and the entirety of the perinatal – the year before and after birth is the site of many such 'catastrophes' – which are intense, emotional, biological and turbulent in rapid waves of succession. But to read such a site of catastrophic change as purely biological and the affective linked solely to such biology is to be blinkered, for these sit within, across and against a range of social structures, as the theorisation of intensive mothering draws attention to. But, as this book argues, all of this unfolds in mediated and increasingly datafied digital societies, where a separation of the social and the digital is untenable (Couldry & Hepp, 2018). Through the *perinatal ideal*, I seek to draw these two literatures together, from sociology and communication studies, to offer me a fruitful lens with which to look at the data I consider in this book.

Mediating early motherhood

Early motherhood and the perinatal in Western societies have witnessed, like possibly all other spheres of life, a rapid and progressive arrival of media and communication technologies into its realm. These have arguably been shaping the ways in which mothers communicate, find information and connect with each other, the ways in which institutions address women and their families, the ways in which healthcare professionals engage with their patients and indeed, the ways in which mediated visual cultures around us, from mainstream media to vlogs to microblogs mediate bodies and maternity. Some aspects of these processes are unwelcome and unjust interruptions, as the recent harvesting and selling of maternal data by Bounty is, symptomatic of life in datafied societies (Das & Ytre-Arne, 2018). Some aspects of these same processes might be regarded as developments in the solely positive sense of the term, for instance, women's self-reported sense of success and satisfaction from online information seeking apps in pregnancy (Lupton et al., 2016), albeit not often critiquing and evaluating these.

But across a wide spectrum of such practices, arguably these processes have been transformative and, like countless other societal processes, early motherhood – in the way it is represented, discussed, experienced, managed, surveiled and sold – is increasingly mediated. Mediation has become central, one might argue, to the way the perinatal and early motherhood is framed in contemporary Western societies. This is not simply, or at all, as a function of what the media does to mothers or what *effect* it has on social actors of the perinatal period in their role as *audiences*, but rather, such centrality has been arrived at by opening up both challenges and possibilities, tools as well as impediments, resources as well as restraints, in the ways in which women and those around them approach, experience and make sense of the perinatal in the contexts of their everyday lives. Under the central umbrella of mediation, one might argue that the perinatal has seen transformative changes in terms of *representations*, in terms of interpersonal *connections* and, whilst this is less relevant to the focus on this particular book but of increasingly overwhelming relevance more broadly – *intrusions* attendant to datafication and the perinatal.

Despite a recent rise in interest in the media and maternity, Downing's comment on the divorce (2008) between media studies and related fields rings true, as a clear account of the mediation of the perinatal is yet to emerge within the growing literature on the mediation of parenting, especially in the context of networked communication. The key word here remains *mediation* – I am interested in the (digital) mediation of early motherhood, with a specific focus on the mediated structures of pressures and struggles women speak about in relation to the perinatal. Mediation beckons us to consider the fundamental roles played by digital communication in making sense of the way the perinatal situates itself in women's lives, including communication between partners, between mothers and midwives, institutions and publics, between mothers and their female relatives, between mothers and other mothers, on anonymous online communities, between television and audiences, between individuals and institutions. Approaching the perinatal through the intellectual lens of mediation makes it crucial to unpack how communication lies at the heart of many of the institutions of the perinatal and the tensions and relationships it represents for individual and institutional actors, as they operate in society contributing to and working with, within and against often competing discourses. This involves an understanding of representations, interpretations, and communication at the levels of individuals acting in relation to domestic partnerships, in relation to families near and far away and in relation to society, culture, media and communication technologies, and the many kinds of private and public institutions involved in all these spheres. Scholars within medical history, the history and sociology of risk in the perinatal and within art history and visual culture studies will locate these against the empirically evidenced series of widespread historical changes in the way the perinatal is approached and experienced, from ancient times to modernity. While this theme of the wider historical transformations to the perinatal falls outside the remits of this book, it is only against that wider temporal and spatial context that we can begin to speak about the mediation of the perinatal most holistically in contemporary societies (see here, Furedi, 2008; Wolf, 2011), as we have begun to see how the 'priceless' infant and the fetal celebrity have become tied to 'good' mothering and the overworked mother. This last – the question of longstanding processes of change in both perinatal processes and in these as the subjects of circulating representations, connections and discourses – can be grasped within the theorisations of mediatisation (Couldry & Hepp, 2018), which posits a meta-theory of the interweaving of media and communication technologies as central institutions in modernity into all other social and political institutions of contemporary societies. This represents a complex project so far as the perinatal is concerned, demanding the long-term participation and collaboration between diverse fields and disciplines, including media studies, health and biological sciences, midwifery, sociology, anthropology, race and migration studies, cultural studies, art history, literature and other areas.

In this book, while I have selected a few digital platforms to focus on in chapters 3 and 4 and in fieldwork which I write out of in chapters 5, 6 and 7, participants were never restricted by either format or platform or genre; our free-flowing conversations were rooted first and foremost in their lived, daily lives and digital technologies – whatever form it took – wove in and out of our conversations, within a framework and approach defined by a focus on mediation. Mediation, for this project, has also not simply been about considering institutionally controlled media (public service television or private television programmes) and user-generated content within an institutional framework (YouTube videos, Facebook groups), but equally about mediated interpersonal communication and the myriad ways in which the two spill into each other. Silverstone's view of mediation as dialectical is particularly central to this task, for it means privileging neither 'the media' nor the audience in making sense of the way meaning is reproduced and circulated within society, including perinatal mothers, other mothers, partners, midwives, other health care organisations and professionals, relatives, friends. This view of mediation presents, texts, interpretation, reception and contexts in a constant interplay where media and communication technologies weave into societal processes and institutions, neither as a cure-all nor as a villain.

Couldry suggests:

> rather than seeing mediation as a dialectic or implied conversation, it may be more productive, I suggest, to see mediation as capturing a variety of dynamics within media flows. By 'media flows', I mean flows

> of production, flows of circulation, flows of interpretation or reception, and flows of recirculation as interpretations flow back into production or flow outwards into general social and cultural life.
>
> (p. 9)

This project never began with people's interpretations of discretely defined texts or made itself entirely about specific texts or formats in particular. An understanding of early motherhood in digital societies must necessarily engage with the question of flows – of meaning, power and communication – where "mediation requires us to understand how processes of communication change the social and cultural environments that support them as well as the relationships that individuals and institutions have to that environment and to each other" (Silverstone, 2002, p. 7). This involves attention to actors and institutions, agency and structure, and addresses the frameworks of reference which are contributed to by mediated communication, which are then mobilised in interpretation and communication by people in their everyday lives. Attendant to this vision of mediation is an understanding of power (see Thompson, 1995), not just of texts to represent, of information and communication technologies to transmit and connect, but also of women as mothers and individuals to access, interpret and communicate within, against and outside of mediated frameworks of reference. These communication practices, like all communication practices, may work to selectively silence and marginalise or highlight and bring to relief the voices and experiences of others, following Thompson's exposition of the management of visibility and the struggle for recognition (1995) in everyday life, both processes intrinsically mediated:

> The visual backdrop to (…) maternal figurations is an unending parade of images of beautiful, young, white, tight pregnant and postpartum celebrity bodies. … The maternal has never been so very public, so hyper visible, but the wall of commentary, which surrounds the maternal and the images that represent it, is deeply incoherent.
>
> (Tyler, 2009, p. 5)

Childbirth potentially has seen the greatest visibility, amidst all things perinatal, and as Tyler and Baraitser (2013) have claimed, birth is visible. This stands against a longer history of reviving interest in maternal bodies and birth in the face of 'matricide', where mothers and birthing bodies were systematically erased in terms of mediated representations. As Tyler remarks above, the last decades have seen a massive proliferation of maternal bodies in the media. Betterton (2009) identifies this appearance to be simultaneously private and public, intimate and displayed, individual and collective. It could, as the previous section has revealed, simultaneously be read as both a vehicle for creative participation with and in the media an expression of agency and choice, and in parallel, a deeply gendered, classed and normative articulation of maternal subjectivities, producing a specific kind of maternal value, embodying an individualised maternal self, in neoliberal times. Tyler and Baraitser's (2013) explorations of the politics of the 'new visibility' of birthing bodies in visual culture is key, for these beckon a deeper engagement than to assume simplistically a linear journey of progress from historic maternal invisibility (see the abundant literature on 'matricide', Baraitser, 2009; Jacobs, 2007, Kristeva, 1989; see also Nash, 2012a, 2012b, on pregnant embodiment) to a new uber-visibility across all forms of mediated communication, demanding critical interrogation of the kinds of maternal subjectivities and in the end, gendered politics that are represented by these new visibilities.

For Tyler and Baraitser, the new genre of Childbirth TV presents a new avatar of the technocratic model of childbirth with women, experiencing a crisis (birth) which needs resolving in medical, hospital-based settings. While drawing from the critical questioning of the technocratic visibility of maternal bodies, one might equally, following scholarship on intensive mothering in relation to infant feeding (Lee, 2008), for instance, query the opposite end of the spectrum, so to speak, of these representations – the all-natural, un-medicalised, almost mythical narratives of birthing within home-made birthing videos, as Mack (2016) elucidates splendidly. Mack's analysis of the mobilising of pain (and the euphoric transcendence of pain) in home-birth videos locates pain to be not just "framed as central to the narrative but also valorized as maternal subjects are depicted enduring, embracing, or even enjoying their encounter with pain" (2016, p. 56). Such small-scale, inexpensive, personally focused media productions celebrating or marking individual accomplishments, journeys and relationships have been at the heart of the Digital Storytelling project (Lambert, 2006). Of importance here is what Friedlander (2008) calls digital narratives' aspiration to speaking about 'a world' rather than simply one text being shared between author and audience. This is achieved through a range of means: "Each of its elements – space, time, objects, beings and actions – can be selected, arranged and transformed for the needs of an aesthetic experience" (2008, p. 186). The multimodal nature (Kress, 2003) of these compositions demarcate them from other maternal compositions, for instance, developed in textual form, even if online (c.f. Pedersen, 2016; Rogers, 2015). They curate an audiovisual world, embedded in digital spaces of sharing, hyper-linking and circulating, in an endless processes of semiosis (Kress, 2003), and these carefully curated stories collectively form parts of the narratives making up a mediated framework of reference (c.f. Silverstone, 1999), which are then accessed and referenced by others about to give birth or those seeking to make sense of their own birthing experiences. The use of these amateur, home-made birthing videos, of course, speaks to the long-discussed participatory potential of new media technologies, at a route to challenging mainstream flows of content (c.f. Burgess & Green, 2013), with the architecture of YouTube built around sharing, commenting, liking, linking, uploading and 'channelling' affording spaces for creative engagement with mediated environments from very small to very large scales. Particularly, however, the concept of curation in this context deserves attention.

While some have spoken of how the architecture of digital technology act as 'curators' holding people's self-representations (c.f. Hogan, 2010), the visual material analysed in the next chapter, for instance, speaks more to the idea of the agency and literacy some birthing women clearly display through very careful strategies of image selection, editing, voicing and composing music in producing very multimodal forms of self-representation towards specific ends, using the technological architectures and toolsets available to them (see also Duffy, 2015, writing on strategic, individualised, self-branding practices). This brings the notion of curation employed here close to what Vivienne and Burgess (2013) have called curated exhibitions of the self. As they go on to note:

> ... tensions are played out and negotiated at the most granular levels of production and distribution; in the material choices the storytellers make as they select, arrange, edit, and manipulate personal images that are combined into relatively stable texts; and in the material decisions they make in sharing these stories with intimate and unknown, as well as sympathetic, indifferent or hostile publics.
>
> (p. 24)

The three features of these narratives which stand out for Couldry (2008) are a pressure to limit duration, standardise the nature of narratives and combine multiple modes such as written text, sound, images. These features do not simply lend themselves to one single logic, but rather, Couldry suggests, involve forms of both presenting and withholding aspects of one's experiences; it is, then, a purposefully curated, mediated narrative, representing selectively, making specific syntactic and semantic choices instead of others. These narratives have critical roles to play in the mediation of social, political and cultural institutions by producing and maintaining hierarchies of voice and power – within which lies their great potential for critique and action and equally, potential for in/exclusion. Couldry identifies the roles of these narratives in the mediation of societal institutions thus:

> When a practice such as digital storytelling challenges media's normal concentration of symbolic resources so markedly, analysing the consequences for wider society and culture is precisely difficult, but it cannot be ignored because of the possibility that digital storytelling is part of a wider democratization, a reshaping of the hierarchies of voice and agency, which characterize mediated democracies.
>
> (2008, p. 11)

Developing a clear picture of the role of mediated communication in the social and biological institutions of early motherhood, as they spill increasingly into contemporary visual cultures (c.f. Locatelli, 2017), requires us to "understand how processes of communication change the social and cultural environments that support them as well as the relationships that individuals and institutions have to that environment and to each other" (Silverstone, 2002, p. 7). This involves attention to actors and institutions, agency and structure, and addresses the frameworks of reference which are contributed to by discourses online, which are then mobilised in interpretation and communication by people in their everyday lives. Of course, images and texts in the world around us, along with a wide variety of other things, resource the kind of expectations and emotions women carry to early motherhood and perinatal experiences. Thinking about birth, while the majority of births in Western industrialised nations 'go well', there are many who leave the moment of birth with lasting trauma and look for support on social media. This is evidenced by pages upon pages of anonymous discussions on parenting websites. Global flows of people mean that practices and advice from cultures of origin often collide with those finding themselves experiencing the perinatal in the West. The contrast (and connection) of cultures and generations is renegotiated by perinatal mothers, using information, advice and support that is constantly mediated. Birth, breastfeeding, weaning, returning or not returning to work are all sometimes idealised or medicalised and, as is evident from the research conducted for this book, too often graded. Tracy Jensen writes valuably about online maternal environments, as she argues that radical and emancipatory possibilities of such spaces often fail to reach their potential because "this assembled potential becomes diffused by the very architecture of the site, which invites mothers into relationships of antagonism, into processes of social distinction and into an individualised and fragmented politics of parenting" (Jensen, 2013, p. 128). A theme which runs through contemporary scholarship on natural, yet less frequently practiced aspects of mothering (see Faircloth, 2010; Lee, 2008; Miller et al., 2007, writing on certain aspects of infant feeding, for instance), is the simultaneity of inclusion and exclusion. Rather than parenting becoming about resource sharing, a certain kind of tribalism, exclusion and selective inclusion happens in the way subgroups form and operate within parenting cultures, generating and drawing from often contrasting discourses and approaches with regard to parenting. This beckons us to pay attention, under the broad umbrella of mediation, not just to representations and circulations of meaning, but to the myriad digitally mediated *connections* mothers establish in negotiating the perinatal and the ways in which these work within and against a variety of resources and restraints.

Chen's critique (2013) of the discourse about mothers blogging links to the wider public derision around women's forums and women's online talk. Chen's techno-feminist critique develops Butler's work on performativity to counter the very rhetoric of 'mommy blogging' (which we can extend to all forms of social media activity that is specific to mothers/parents) to stress that the terminology itself reinforces women's roles as nurturers alone and puts women in a box, so to speak. While Chen links this to ideal mother prototypes, I argue that the 'mommy terminology' (instead of mother, for example) works also as a convenient, ready-to-employ device of light-hearted dismissal of these texts as anything to be seriously taken or analysed. Part of this may well link to the commercialisation of these spaces as Hunter (2016) in her recent study argues, but there is a broader debate to be had about the words we use to refer to women's/mothers' textual practices on social media.

Rogers (2015) offers 'maternal essayists' as a new category of mothers writing online. Her focus is on the narrative techniques, artistic self-expression and negotiations of agency by mothers in online communication as they speak of their own lives and stories. Rogers is interested in "how digital representations reflect and help define or (re)shape the realities of women and families, and how mothering and being a mother are political, personal and creative narratives unfolding within the digital world" (p. 248). Her account is particularly poignant because it pays attention to the fine twists and turns of writing, reminding us to pay attention to the important details in such writing through which voice and identity is mediated that we might often not notice as we mine the Web for vast volumes of data. She reminds us of the value of this writing, as it depicts "the ways in which mothering and being a mother are political, personal and creative narratives unfolding within the digital world" (p. 259), something Lopez (2009) positions as a radical act, and Morrison (2011) as the grounds for an 'intimate public' to become visible.

As Dahlen and Homer's (2013) work has shown, the texts collectively created on online platforms become a lens into broader societal discourses around parenting, birth, children and indeed, the philosophies through and within which life experiences and aspirations are formed and framed. Pettigrew et al. found in 2015 that the maintenance of social ties and managing of stress related with parenting underlies the social media practices of mothers. These included, for them, the "developing connections with others, experiencing heightened levels of mental stimulation, achieving self-validation, contributing to the welfare of others, and extending skills and abilities" (p. 510). These resonate closely also with Chen's findings recently (2015) that engagement, information and recreation play key roles in this process. The Cyberparents project looked at mothers using online forums for advice on their children's health and also transitioning into motherhood. The conclusions were clear there that online support merges with and complements offline support in this regard (O'Connor & Madge, 2004, p. 351). The same scholars found a few years earlier that "the internet was both liberating and constraining: it played an important social role for some women while at the same time it encouraged restrictive and unequal gender stereotypes in this particular community of practice" (Madge and O'Connor, 2006, p. 199). Johnson (2015) terms these websites 'intimate mothering publics' which she suggests "are particularly useful for thinking about the meaning-making practices and learning experiences that occur during intimate online and face-to-face interactions" (p. 237). Chan's (2008) account of virtual space and motherhood in Hong Kong reinforces that these forums develop beyond their "technology-mediated nature into a community of face-to-face friendships and social and emotional support" (p. 169). And yet, these are also spaces where discourses of 'good motherhood' are constructed and performed, as Cheresheva discovers in her recent (2015) study on online narratives of infant feeding in Hungary and Bulgaria (see also Cappellini & Yen, 2016; Gray, 2013).

I turn specifically, now, to the work around interpersonal connections online. Amidst the querying of enthusiasm around digital health on the one hand (Harvey, 2016; Koteyko et al., 2015) and the lack of a distinct space for maternal digital well-being on the other in larger Digital Health plans in the U.K., this book suggests that we bring together a repertoire of concepts as lenses to look at the contextualised, complex and nuanced ways in which perinatal relationships are digitally mediated. Interpersonal relationships in computer-mediated environments have long been studied from a range of sociological, psychological and socio-cultural perspectives. One strand of evidence has considered, over time, how online social ties compare to offline ones, in terms of outcomes. Here, as sociological studies of the internet noted early on (c.f. Haythornthwaite, 2002; Wellman et al., 1996), computer-mediated environments were often thought to be providing a reduced-cues form of communication, often considered, as Baym (2015) notes, to be inferior to face-to-face communication, although these were also considered to be useful and integrative (Jones, 1998; Smith & Kollock, 1999).

While academic evidence in this regard has historically split between findings that digitally mediated ties bring positive or less than positive consequences (White & Dorman, 2001), evidence on friendships, intimacy, trust and social support of diverse kinds shows a range of generally positive outcomes (Amichai-Hamburger et al., 2007). These are particularly clear for stigmatised social groups or those seeking social support for particular health conditions (c.f. Amichai-Hamburger & Furnham, 2007; Wellman & Gulia, 1999) and those seeking and providing comforting communication and empathy (c.f. Caplan & Turner, 2007). A second key strand of findings has considered the role of self-disclosure online. Self-disclosure, in the rich literature on mediated intimacies, has been known to be the engine that drives intimacies (Chambers, 2013). Evidence shows here that anonymity, pseudonimity, homophily, freedom from geographical boundaries and control over when one can leave the conversation offer implications for higher amounts of self-disclosure and trust online, shaping the formation of online ties considerably (Amichai-Hamburger et al., 2013). A third strand of work has considered how online and offline ties compare in terms of interactional quality, nature and process. Here it has been posited that the nature of social ties differs between online and offline interactions, with digitally mediated relationships generally emerging to support weaker social ties, that is, "loose connections between individuals who may provide useful information or new perspectives for one another but typically not emotional support" (Ellison et al., 2007).

But the boundaries between online and offline social ties, risks and opportunities presented by these ties (c.f. Valkenburg & Peter, 2011) and their benefits and drawbacks have long been evidenced to be far from watertight. Online relationships often move offline (Baym, 2015), and strong ties in offline relationships show significant amounts of online facets.

Madianou and Miller's conceptualisation of *polymedia* in this context (2012) brings work on interpersonal relationships into direct dialogue with the now established understanding in media and communication studies that communication technologies themselves and societal processes can no longer be delinked. They also posit that mediated interactions and relationships involve ethical, moral and emotional choices made in mediated communication, out of an entire mediasphere as a connected whole rather than as individual technical interfaces. Fascinating recent research on *mediated intimacies* (Petersen et al., 2017) shows how these digitally mediated relationships and intimacies can also perform regulative functions. Andreassen (2017) states that producing and maintaining normative understandings of family and family roles, prompt an understanding of these intimacies at the intersection of individual agency and societal structure. Intimacy itself has been co-constituted and transformed through the arrival of networks with social media involved in the private and public display of emotions and self-disclosure (Chambers, 2013). Davies (2017) contends that these mediated intimacies are simultaneously very personal but still retain a public character.

Cutting across these conversations about circulating representations of perinatality, the study of networked, mediated connections of perinatality and the physical, emotional and social aspects of parenting (c.f. Gong, 2016), the increasing arrival and uptake of what Mollen and Dhaenens (2018) term intrusive interfaces beckon particular attention. This is particularly key at a time when much writing about parenthood focuses on the parenting of older children and teenagers, and does not often include similar accounts of the mediation of pregnancy, birthing, infant feeding, postnatal mental health difficulties, sleep, weaning and the myriad experiences of parenting and motherhood in infancy and very early childhood. The rise of interest in datafication is actively changing this last and welcome interventions are arriving to populate this field (c.f. Barassi, 2017; Locatelli, 2017, amongst others; Mascheroni, 2018). Tiidenberg and Baym (2017) elucidate, for instance, the performance of pregnancy akin to Tyler and Baraitser's body project (2013) on online spaces, whilst an array of digital footprints of 4D and 3D scans are invited by a mushrooming of commercial providers, inviting the sharing and recording of these for posterity (Leaver & Highfield, 2016). Barassi's excellent account of pregnancy apps (2017) draws attention to some of the complexities of these apps and their meanings in specific socio-cultural contexts of sharing, connecting, risk perception and identity work. While a large part of this work sits within conversations on infants, parental surveillance, monitoring and policing the bodies of those without a voice yet worthy of critique equally are these interfaces themselves in terms of the self-surveilling engagement they invite (Lupton, 2017) from mothers, the recirculation of idealised mother-child bonds and unity they make discursively apparent and the costs of these intrusions to women, as they function, amidst the gendered contexts of intensive motherhood.

The perinatal ideal

This book concerns itself with these mediated communicative relationships around the perinatal as well as social structures which shape early motherhood and the many messy emotions involved in the sort of rhetoric, pressures, struggles, exclusions and inclusions this book speaks about. But it argues fundamentally that the two are inseparable, and one is incomplete without attention to the other if one is to consider the ways in which perinatality functions in contemporary digital societies. To bring these two foregoing bodies of work together, I draw upon the notion of *the perinatal ideal*. I think of the perinatal ideal as a mediated ideology which functions at the intersections of the specific biological and sociological nature of the intensity of the perinatal period and the myriad gendered, structural pressures it entails, and the proliferation and uptake of newer platforms and devices circulating an array of discourses, rhetoric, connections, disconnections and newer practices of sharing and surveilling. I conceptualise the perinatal ideal as an individualising, responsibilising, morally weighted, mediated and deeply affective set of conditions which traverses a multitude of objects and spaces to produce and maintain the very conditions of early mother in digital societies. Located firmly within the intensive motherhood ideology (Hays, 1998), it derives its specificity from the particular conditions of the perinatal. These particularities derive from the unique rapidity of infant development which occurs in the first year post-birth and the concentrated, critical and amplified interfaces with policy and practice institutions and individuals involved with infant well-being and healthcare that mothers must engage with, and ever-increasing technological advancement that parents, but particularly mothers, are invited to take up and take part in.

In such a mediated context of intensive mothering, the perinatal ideal is cause and effect, condition and outcome, discourse and materiality. It embeds the mediation of the perinatal in the sociology of neo-liberal motherhood (c.f. Jensen & Tyler, 2012; Littler, 2013; McRobbie, 2013; Tyler, 2011). I have discussed in this chapter the need for mothers to be self-disciplining subjects (Gill, 2007; McRobbie, 2009), as evident in the strongly classed 'deviancy' debates around good and bad mothering (c.f. Jensen & Tyler, 2012). Attendant to this is a gradation of maternal self-perception, including sensations of not being enough, as it comes across in the many instances in this book. Likewise, the perinatal ideal makes itself manifest and apparent in the production of the maternal self as a subject of value in 'mommy wars' (c.f. Abetz & Moore, 2018) frequently pitched as 'cat fights' – mother fighting mother – in the popular press. Crucially, none of these phenomena can be effectively understood at the level of the individual mother.

The notion of the perinatal ideal rests clearly on feminist sociological work around motherhood and mothering, as this chapter has outlined. From Kristeva and Goldhammer's theorisation of primary narcissism in 'Stabat mater' (1985), which refers to the seemingly unproblematic unity of mother and child, Arendt's work on natality to theorisations of political, economic and cultural imperatives in contemporary Western societies on mothers to be intensively tied to their infants (c.f. Faircloth, 2013), imperatives to perform 'good mothering' in perinatal years link clearly and overtly to intensive mothering (Sharon Hays, 1998; see also Wolf, 2011). The perinatal ideal finds particular context and meaning in relation to contemporary socio-historical shifts in the division of childcare-related labour at every phase of the perinatal and beyond. Harman and Capellini (2015) write, for instance, on children's lunchboxes as a site of interaction between family practices and institutions, which sits against the context of the political, economic and cultural logics of neo-liberalism (Bochantin et al., 2010; Moravec, 2011; O'Brien Hallstein, 2011). British sociological scholarship has had considerable significance here (c.f. Jensen & Tyler, 2012; Littler, 2013; McRobbie, 2013; Tyler, 2011), critiquing the political-economic and cultural contexts within which "maternal subjectivities are produced and maintained and mother blame and guilt rationalized, as an individualized, idealized maternal subjectivity privileged within the intensive motherhood discourse" (Das, 2018). Such work has questioned the unproblematic unity of mother and child (both as an infant and as a fetus, relevant for a discussion on the perinatal, which both precedes and succeeds the appearance of the child as an individual), celebrating the inseparability of mother and child as the maternal ideal with narratives of the perinatal critiqued, for instance, by Parker (1997) in terms of how perinatal change and development is conceptualised only in terms of the child and not the mother, ignoring maternal 'labour' involved in gendered norms of care-related responsibilities and burdens in the very early years (Ruddick, 1994). In addition, as mentioned previously, these burdens are experienced differentially, and perinatal mental well-being is also experienced with an array of additional complexities among migrant and minority ethnic communities. Feminist geographical work, particularly the limited work that exists on natality and migration (c.f. Gedalof, 2009), has complicated the dualities of connection/disconnection, travelling/staying put, querying the assumption of large networks of offline familial support as being necessarily positive (Ryan, 2011).

But such sociological frameworks are not enough, I suggest, to fully grasp what is going on with the perinatal in a mediated social world. These very discourses of mother blame, maternal erasure, maternal responsibilisation operate in a world which is inherently polymedia (Madianou & Miller, 2012), where conditions of deep mediatisation (Couldry & Hepp, 2018) make it impossible to separate the social and the digital. These, then, are conditions where we cannot possibly understand the formation of peer relationships in communities of mothers struggling with perinatal depression, for instance, or the range of exclusive and inclusive discourses circulating on online perinatal communities without grasping the way online interpersonal ties (Baym, 2015; Das, 2018) function. These, then, are conditions where we cannot make sense of mother blame and maternal responsibilisation without unpacking conditions of dataveillance (Van Dijck, 2013), where inviting the maternal gaze inwards to monitor herself and her infant lubricate the very systems and structures through which we live in conditions of surveillance and monitoring. Such conditions make it impossible to make sense of the critical role of self-disclosure and the formation of intimacies without understanding these as networked intimacies (Andreassen et al., 2017) or the role of disclosure online (Amichai-Hamburger et al, 2013). Such conditions of mediation mean turning our attention to the perinatal ideal as not simply a sociological notion, but by definition a mediated one, where "social actors continue to pursue their social ends but mediated through digital interfaces" (Couldry & Hepp, 2016, p. 1).

3 The *good* birth[1]

In this chapter, I begin to take a look at the perinatal ideal as a mediated, responsibilising ideology, by focusing on *representations* of birthing in amateur, home-made video productions. I look at the ways in which agentic engagement with technological architecture and multimodal forms of curation and creation feed into and out of discourses around the intensive perinatal and the all-sacrificing mother that my discussions of the perinatal ideal in Chapter 2 have alluded to. What makes representations of childbirth particularly fascinating as a site of analysis for the perinatal ideal is the juxtaposition of two discourses. One is the emancipatory, feminist revival of women asserting themselves against the white-coated, often male, medical community, harking back to the natural birthing movement in the U.S.A. and U.K. (Gaskin, 2003; Kitzinger, 2012a). The other is the neo-liberal, self-regulating, self-managing, highly individualised discourse of ideal births and ideal birthing modes which derive out of the intensive motherhood discourse (Hays, 1998), which Chapter 2 alluded to in discussing the perinatal ideal. My central argument in this chapter and the one that follows is that rather than seeing them as competing discourses, it is more productive to consider 'natural' birth and by extension, women's representations of birthing on social media as a coin of which these two discourses represent two sides. My findings consistently show across these platforms, a mix of positive and less than positive nuancing of birth and birthing-related discourse. Chapter 4 shows, for instance, how online discussions offer a cathartic, empowering and questioning space, as women prepare for and make sense of childbirth. In contrast, they also often work to silence and shut down as 'horror stories' experiences which do not fit into narratives of 'good' birthing.

Before I present my analysis, I would like to locate this chapter within the specific context of the U.K., where the hypnobirthing movement could be said to have spread to from the vastly different medical cultures from many other Western nations, for instance, the U.S.A. Free at the point of use healthcare, provided by the National Health Service, means that the overwhelming majority of births in the U.K. do not happen with either private medical providers or private health insurance. NHS-led settings, which include home births with NHS midwives, or midwife-led births at birth centres or, if need be, consultant-led hospital births, cover the vast majority of births in the U.K., where most mothers use NHS free at the point of use services for birth and postnatal care. The NHS message, along with the message from the leading childbirth charity in the U.K. – the National Childbirth Trust – is very supportive of un-intervened births. In my fieldwork for this book, I conducted interviews with mothers, where some have cited the pressure on public services as reasons they may not have received pain relief on time despite opting for it, and equally, women who have asked for more support for un-intervened births or establishing breastfeeding have felt that they have had to struggle to find easily available resources. This, in the context of austerity measures in the recent years, also ties in with other kinds of pressures on health services which are meant to be supporting mothers perinatally. A discussion of these austerity-related struggles on the British National Health Service ties in with the question of maternal choice and agency which is discussed further in Chapter 7. In the U.K., the Royal College of Midwives (2014) note, "neither midwives nor maternity support workers feel they have enough time to deliver the emotional health care that women need and deserve" (p. 11). This is echoed by a recent BBC report, "only 3% of NHS local commissioning groups had a postnatal mental health strategy" (BBC, 2016) and support works currently on a "postcode lottery in which two in three women currently affected missed out on vital help" (*The Guardian*, 2016). Online forums – including video sharing sites, microblogs, Facebook groups and parenting sites are rapidly becoming 24/7, anonymous sources of support, in the face of a system under pressure. And precisely thus, the rhetorical strategies, devices and 'ideological weight' of the kinds of maternal subjectivities mediated on these platforms deserve critical attention, for these form part of the mediated frameworks of reference which women use as lenses with which to position and interpret their own lives, choices and experiences.

In discussing this project with both lay and elite members of the public outside the field of media and communication studies, particularly in conversations with those in the sector of women's health and healthcare in general, and with mothers themselves, I have been reminded multiple times that it is high time one studied the 'effects' of the media on birthing women. This has usually come from two different directions. One has contended that the media has hyper-medicalised childbirth and the other has contended that the media has created unrealistic pressures on birthing women to get birth 'right'. Both have reminded me that this is the media *effect* this project needs to establish. This continues to be an attractive idea in the public domain – the effect of the media on any political, social or cultural institution or process is always, perhaps, guaranteed to be a conversation peg, when in reality, the development of the field of media and communication studies has seen the development of the theorising of mediation as opposed to the effect of the media *on* something. This has meant a massive shift of focus from direct effects of the media, through empirical evidencing of audience activity, towards a more long-term interest in the ways in which the media is intrinsically woven into processes in society, thereby fundamentally reshaping constantly the ways in which these processes develop and function.

So, videos I consider in this chapter might prompt us to think what they represent, that is, do they represent something more than the specific values of a distinct natural birthing community, and if so what is it and why? Equally, one could fruitfully analyse how ubiquitous they are or not, how many people view them, how pervasive they are for instance and what sort of conversations materialise around them. In this chapter, however, my focus is specifically on curating and representing meaning as I consider the skilful use of multimodal repertoires to produce visual cultures through which a highly specific maternal subjectivity is mediated. These visual cultures draw upon fundamentals of the *intensive* perinatal, as elucidated in my discussion of the perinatal ideal. This includes the abjection of maternal subjects (Tyler & Baraithser, 2013), an enormity of maternal labour (Parker, 2005) and the subsequent rise of the hyper-mediated new maternal visibility and its own cultural politics of positioning the neo-liberal maternal self, transcending all pain, within the intensive motherhood discourse (Bochantin et al., 2010; Douglas & Michaels, 2005; Hays, 1996; O'Brien Hallstein, 2011). Part of the work on maternal selves can be traced back to earlier roots in Kristeva's theorisation (1989) of primary narcissism and the seemingly unproblematic unity of mother and child, to Arendt's work on natality (1958), to Butler's work on gender and performativity (1997) and to more recent work in communication and cultural studies by Gill and Orgad (2016) and McRobbie (2009) on the neo-liberal maternal self. This work has begun, as I write, with Tyler and Baraithser's attention to the visual cultures of birth (2013), De Benedictis's work on the reception of the television show One Born Every Minute (2017), Mack's (2016) work on home births and a network in the U.K. on Televising Childbirth, as this work was produced.

The YouTube case

This case studied amateur YouTube videos portraying a specific style of natural births called hypnobirths, which make use of relaxation and hypnosis techniques during labour and birthing, and offer an alternative to birthing in interventionist, obstetrics-led settings. Following Mack (2016), it is important to note here, however, the term 'natural' birth itself is loaded and that "the use of the term natural to describe home birth or unmedicated vaginal birth is highly contested. The term, some have argued, denotes that other forms of birth are unnatural, wrong, or inherently problematic" (p. 64). Hypnobirthing has developed into a widespread system of actors, objects and institutions, including classes teaching relaxation exercises, the availability of extensive study material, practice exercises with partners, infographics, nature-inspired 'positive' imagery, renowned teachers and practitioners, year-round courses, online courses, certifications, online forums, Facebook groups, Twitter hashtags, a very wide selection of professional and home videos on sites like YouTube and books. On the one hand, there are visible advantages of relaxation and hypnosis-related birthing support within the context of the natural birthing movement to restore women's agency in birthing, resisting and rejecting hyper-medicalised technocratic cultures of births. But on the other, this chapter suggests that these home-made, amateur hypnobirthing videos need to be viewed against the feminist critique of the *intensive motherhood* discourse, which sees the videos producing the birthing mother as an individualised, self-regulating and highly invested subject, transcending pain in a mythic journey of blissful birthing. The labours of these maternal subjects evident in the carefully curated visuals of the ultimate joyful, painless birth, complete with its own distinct vocabulary that scripts a specific narrative of birth, contribute to mediated frameworks of reference which establish hierarchies of good and bad births, ultimately going against the core feminist critique of technocratic birthing cultures, the very framework they seek to resist. This, of course, is notwithstanding the genuine investment, emotional and physical, these mothers feel and display in the production of these videos. These videos speak to the dichotomy that is increasingly evident around discussions of maternal choice in childbirth and the exclusivity of the heavily gendered dialogue that exists in contemporary Western societies about all-natural, intensive motherhood (c.f. Hays, 1998; see also Smith-Rosenberg & Rosenberg, 1973), starting before conception and extending many years into children's lives, which falls, albeit following a vastly different route, into the same trap, challenging women's choice and agency which we saw within over-medicalised birthing cultures.

To select videos for this project I used search terms such as hypnobirth or hypnobirthing on YouTube and sorted results based on viewership ratings. I selected a subset of 100 videos, most of which had been posted by mothers in the U.K. I note though that it is methodologically significant that I watched many more videos than the 100 selected for the project (only a few of which are used as illustrative instances in what follows). I watched the videos multiple times, following a pen and chapter method of coding, which felt far more comfortable to me in this particular study than computer-assisted coding, and I watch these from beginning to end, multiple times, making notes on these. I paid particular attention to videos with higher viewing figures, as I was keen to find out how far these videos had started travelling. All the videos were analysed using established resources from within visual methodology which provides frameworks for analysing visual texts. Visual methodology is a diverse field with a multiplicity of disciplinary perspectives. This work has been inspired particularly by Theo Van Leeuwen and Cary Jewitt's approach (2001) to the analysis of multimodal visual cultures which incorporates Lister and Wells' (2008) location of images and products of visual culture within a 'circuit of culture' (Du Gay, 1997). This, for them, entails asking a range of questions which move away from locating visual cultures within the boundaries of its frames. These questions include asking where the image is situated in its context, for context shapes expectations; it means asking how the audiences/viewer is invited to engage with the content, including what discourses are authored to appeal most to the viewer. This also involves asking questions of the contexts of production of the content, including the convergence of intention, knowledge and skill. The other aspect they pay attention to is two uses of the concept of conventions within a visual representation – one from within literary and art historical sources and the other from sociological sources. The former draws attention to the materiality of the medium at hand and a recognition of the interpretive role of the viewer in drawing meaning from representations.

The visual logics of mediated hypnobirths

A few key principles stand out across all the videos analysed, which are expanded on in what follows. First, hypnobirthing is ritualised and presented as a near-mythic journey through carefully chosen visual and audio aids, making use of textual devices to create a narrative of not the endurance of pain, but the erasure of it, producing birth not through the pain of labour, but rather as a journey that is ecstatic in going beyond pain at all. Second, sound plays a critical role in the majority of videos, not simply through the addition of it (sound effects, music, instrumental music, fade-ins and outs and other audio editing techniques), but equally through the selective deletion of it (the deletion of any sound which may have indicated discomfort or difficulty felt in the natural course of giving birth). This ties in to the disappearance, rhetorically and visually, of pain – which is of critical significance in the narrative curated by these videos. Third, obscuration in general is significant, be it the blurring of faces, extended fade-outs, selective use of darkness and darkening techniques and as above, often the removal and editing out of vocalisation beyond what seems apparently permissible through faint groaning, sounding close to ecstasy (see my point about the mythic nature of the journey represented through these videos).

In Video M the opening sequence involves a bright, silver starburst that rotates on the screen with uplifting music, erupting into glittery stars – white on black, light on darkness. Multimodal communication helps mediate the narrative in Video M to produce the hypnobirth as a ritualistic experience of the mother who has prepared and practiced to not endure, but overcome any modicum of pain. This is achieved as much by the addition of visual and audio devices as by the textual removal and erasure of experiences, for instance, the darkening, obscuration or non-inclusion of any difficult moments in labour or the removal and editing out of vocalisations.

Sound and voice of the actors (for instance, regular conversation at a birth centre) is removed in Video M, to be replaced with calm, gentle music, creating (selectively) an ambience of peace, quiet and gentle labour, when, in reality, the text does not convey any of the actual sounds in the room at that particular point in the video because the audio tracks have been replaced with pre-edited music and voiceovers, overlaid by text. In Video P, devices like soft focus, very slow zooming in on to the mother's pregnant belly, slowed down breathing, elimination of all natural noises, words and sounds, wide-angle views that look in from the outside into a room where the birthing mother lies, produces, in attendance to the fading in of powerful instrumental music, the narrative of the gentle, calm birth. It is critical to investigate the syntactic and semantic features here, to make sense of how conventions are made use of, created and broken to produce a specific maternal subjectivity.

Both Video M and P are illustrations of how almost every hypnobirthing video analysed for this project could be worked back to literary and art historical approaches to the use of visual conventions which beckon us to pay attention to YouTube and the home-edited video as media, whose materiality is critical in the stories which are created and carried on them. Video Y makes use of photographic conventions which utilise black and white still photography and near-still videography, with transcendental music, text and the interplay of light and dark to produce a birth video which eliminates any real sounds, colours or shades which one might expect in an 'amateur' home video. Instead, the video is far from amateur. Camera, gaze, lighting, position and context have all been made artistic and well-thought out use of, which, sociologically speaking of course, carry what Lister and Wells (2008) call 'ideological weight'. The use of conventions in this way mediates multimodally (Kress, 2003), an image of the enduring mother who has transcended pain and discomfort – who is at one with nature, and yet, the constant interplay of edited music, edited audio, carefully edited photography and the use of text overlays produces a very intentional narrative. As Friedlander notes (2008), in digital storytelling "thoughts can become visible, objects can metamorphose, according to emotional and aesthetic rules and background elements (such as floors and skies) can suddenly communicate symbolic meaning" (p. 186). This communication of symbolic meaning through the use of photographic and videographic conventions in both shooting and editing is precisely the nature of the visual logic in these hypnobirthing videos. Video F is an instance where the mother diarises her thoughts – again, selectively represented, about the ecstatic process that the birth will be – smiling and speaking through uplifting music and soft focus shots of floral arrangements around a bath which can barely be seen. It is critical that we approach these visual products as a work-in-progress lens into the ideologically weighty discourses shaped, resourced and privileged by the producers, which then enter the circuits of a mediated communicative framework.

What ties these forms of multimodal representations of personal narratives together is what Couldry (2008) calls "a common logic (...) a distinctive 'media logic', that is consistently channeling narrative in one particular direction" (p. 9). This direction, I argue, is taken through the conscious use of careful, multimodal curation in these videos, which demands a certain kind of artistic intent, skill and material possessions. These audiovisual narratives produce birthing mothers as near-mythic heroines through the use of specific textual devices. These heroines go on, usually in silence, with the exception of very soft moans of usually ecstasy, to birth without sound, without pain, without discomfort and in absolute harmony with the rhythmic beats of the music the video is produced with. The media logic (Couldry, 2008) here is that these conventions produce a very selective, heavily edited version of a deeply individualised subject who has prepared with inner work, months of practice with audio tapes that ascribe meaning to natural objects and who has controlled any modicum of pain in labour simply, it seems, by 'letting go'. I argue later in Chapter 4 that difficult birth experiences can often be silenced in anonymous, online discussions – and these all form part of a cultural imaginary which increasingly mediates mothers as intensive, all-enduring, neo-liberal subjects, who are indistinguishable from their infants and who do things 'right' by doing the most natural, organic, absolute best they possibly can. This leads on, from the discussions of visual conventions above to the key narrative of 'goodness' in birthing, which is created through these videos.

'Good birthing'

One of the overwhelming findings from this work has been the 'good birth' – a visual curation of the idyllic and ideal circumstances and forms that a good birth comes with. The narrative around how good the birth is when hypnobirthing draws most clearly from the emphasis on calm and quiet, the use of visuals and imagery to invite visions of nature and natural surroundings, and the use of music and audio editing to produce the hypnobirth as the good birth and the birthing woman as having achieved the ultimate in the entry to motherhood. This finding sits alongside critical feminist theorisations of women doing the 'right' thing in motherhood and from the literature on bad and good parenting and mothering (Yadlon, 1997), including critiques of how normative and exclusionary this heavily gendered discourse can get. In Video A, the mother is clearly experiencing contractions, as evident from her breathing, but she does not mention either the word contraction or pain, calling these 'surges' things that are 'exciting' her, as she beams and smiles while very clearly experiencing physical discomfort. While Mack's (2016) critique of home birth videos analyse pain via the device of masochism in neo-liberal modernity, my findings from hypnobirthing reveal the erasure, overt and covert, of the very word 'pain' itself. By derecognising pain, and indeed forbidding the use of the word pain as in the rest of hypnobirthing discourse, the fundamental physical sensation that accompanies birth is replaced with words like ecstasy, joyful surges or rhythmic sensations, and the feeling of pain is removed from normalcy and positioned as something which needs to be and indeed can be avoided through conscious preparation and choice – birth simply needs to be done right. Visual management is a critical part of documenting this for public view, as in Video C, like in most videos, a hypnosis tape runs in the background, as the mother is shown lying in her bath, with dimmed lighting draping her torso, and the rest of the room in darkness. The grandmother, midwife and partner, at their very supportive best, also appear on the video, encouraging her to bear the 'surges' for what is to come is 'totally worth it'.

In Video D, the mother is described as a 'trooper' as the audio tape encourages her to conquer the surges (never contractions) with her breathing, imagining the colours of the rainbow arching across the sky. These videos amount to much more than, and mostly, never, the emergence of a baby from a birth canal, for it curates a specific narrative of how birth is meant to be done; the preparations involved in listening to and rehearsing with an audio tape are evident as the tape weaves through the video. In Video A, text overlays tell us the story as the story was designed to be told – for the difficulties encountered in the actual crowning and birth of the baby are omitted. The overlaid text at the end, which is laid on to uplifting music, casually alludes to how there were problems with the baby's positioning and some 'help' was needed in getting the baby out; but these are never shown as part of the video, whose sole representation of the birth is near silent sighing in an equally calm and almost silent surrounding. The story which is told in these videos need to be seen as components of a hyper-mediated and readily available narrative, which has been selectively represented to both contribute to and draw from a clearly established normative account of the good birth. The conclusions of most of these videos represent a music-laden, noise and commotion-free birth, one that could so easily be aspired for.

This, on the one hand, works as the rebuttal of over-medicalised settings where choice and agency could be removed from women, but these also work their way into the cultural imaginary to become standards for self-critique. The conclusions often make powerful use of still imagery, with fade-ins and outs, very slow zooming in, professional baby photography aids such as feathers, headbands, soft colourful fabrics and close-ups. Still imagery makes a resounding finale, a grand conclusion, overlaid with uplifting music tracks to create a happy, fulfilled, mother-and-baby moment. It is necessary to critically investigate how these rejections of technocratic birthing cultures produce mythically inflected narratives that offer up carefully curated 'lay' perspectives on maternal subjectivities. These achieve the 'good birth', as they promote endurance, self-governance, sacrifice, selflessness and an individualised narrative of maternity which keeps reproducing and glorifying intensive and all-natural mothering, all explored extensively in the literature developed over the years on the gendered politics of motherhood

(Badinter, 2012; Lee, 2008; amongst others). Attendant to this is the 'moral weight' of birthing, which, as Longhurst (2009b) notes, makes it "important, therefore, to be seen both in 'real' space and cyber/space as doing it 'right', that is, doing it with love, tenderness and care" (p. 93).

Discussion

Of course, these videos might be said to belong to a specific style of natural birthing and as such, we might conclude that their influence or viewership is limited. An analysis of their viewership, or an account of the engagement that results online around them or discussing these with the audiences of these videos would be a fruitful next step. But despite these videos belonging to a specific style and persuasion in relation to natural births, they mobilise discourses, repertoires and metaphors of maternal sacrifice, maternal responsibility and the individualised transcending of pain, which are integral to the perinatal ideal and the way in which mother is framed and positioned in a wide array of child-related conversations, to create the best possible outcomes for the priceless child. As such, these videos need to be located as visualised birthing cultures which spill outside the boundaries framing their material forms. They are to be shared, made into shortened clips, shared on Facebook groups, watched in anticipation by a group of first-time parents who may either have paid a small fortune for a class, or who may not be able to afford a class and might thus be gathering free resources or watched by those who have had traumatic birthing experiences who might then muse about what they did 'wrong' for their own births. These visual cultures contribute to and draw from discourses around childbirth, which include both the overly medicalised ones that deny women agency and those that create the all-enduring, sacrificing ultimate mother who will bear everything with a smile on her face. The context of these videos almost always includes a caring and present partner, usually other family members who are part of the big day, and by default the context also involves a certain level of economic resources and digital skills to create the product that these videos become. The videos therefore emerge out of a confluence of the intent, knowledge and skill, as Lister and Wells pointed out, to curate digital stories. The viewer is invited to engage with the videos from a place of aspiration largely, to know, yes, they can, indeed birth 'well', they too can eliminate 'pain' and welcome a 'surge' instead. There is a subtle and selective choosing of discourses which are written into the videos to appeal most to the viewer. The materiality of YouTube is crucial – it allows for the creating of channels, which can then be followed, commented on, shared and made to be both private and public at will, and they demand not very advanced digital skills to master. Adapting Couldry's questions (2008) about the role played by digital narratives in wider, mediated, communicative frameworks, these maternal embodiments online, created, curated, maintained, using a range of artistic and aesthetic tools, beg a range of questions. In what ways do these narratives of good births include and exclude? What are the long-term consequences of these audiovisual practices online which represent a very specific narrative of childbirth? How do these representations of the maternal, simultaneously public and private, yet inherently selective, bear critical consequences for the highly mediated institution of childbirth?

A large component and product of the good-bad discourse mobilised within the perinatal ideal is blame and guilt. Elliott et al. (2015) locate the roots of blame and guilt within the discourse of intensive motherhood: "if – as the ideology of intensive mothering posits – mothers are ultimately responsible for and capable of ensuring their children's wellbeing, then they are also to blame for any problems their children encounter" (p. 367). Blame has a key role to play in the context of the perinatal ideal, with failing to perform according to these standards resulting in self-blame and guilt (Barnes & Power, 2015), and blame being placed on 'failing' mothers by the popular press and institutions. This last is poignantly captured by Orgad and De Benedictis' (2015) content analysis of media coverage of stay-at-home mothers, which probes further into the seemingly illogical (in neo-liberal terms) praise allocated to mothers who sacrifice their professions and careers, opting out as economic actors to stay at home. The logic they find is in a focused rehearsing and reinforcing of traditional gender roles, whereby these sacrifices (presented as worthy) make the male of the household capable of becoming ultra-productive. The stay-at-home mother, who speaks often of her 'choices', is then a neo-liberal subject, as evident from their analysis (Gill & Orgad, 2016, writing on 'confidence cultures' in girls; Littler, 2013, p. 227, writing about the "conservative fantasy of autonomous, individualizing retreatism" of 'yummy mummies' and Akass, 2012 on motherhood and myth-making). Childcare is a particularly relevant site for the study of intensive motherhood, as McRobbie's analysis of contemporary British motherhood reveals (2009) where conservative popular discourse has systematically constructed the intensively hands-on (yet suitably 'feminine') mother, staying at home, as the ideal of intensive (and desirable) motherhood, which in itself is part of a broader project of framing parenting as project of reflexive individualisation with the attendant production of value (see De Benedictis, 2012, on 'feral' parenting; also Gajjala, 2015, on digital labour and new domesticity).

As I argue in the next chapter, two cross-cutting discourses blurring issues of agency, control and power have emerged with regard to the now heavily mediated birthing body – a finding which applies to the visual logics of mediated hypnobirthing explored in this chapter as well. If real feminist agency located within and through the emancipatory, feminist revival of women asserting themselves against the white-coated, often male, medical community, harking back to the introduction of the natural birthing movement in the U.S.A. and U.K. (Gaskin, 2003; Kitzinger, 2012a), foregrounded the critical importance of women's voices in the labour room, the more recent neo-liberal, self-regulating, self-managing, highly individualised discourse of ideal births and ideal birthing modes which sit within the intensive motherhood discourse (Hays, 1998) swings the pendulum, it seems, so far as to constrain that very agency. While medicalised discourses, encouraging cultures of fear and anxiety around birthing typically remove women's control, hypnobirthing discourses emphasise women's control, and indeed near-mythical victory over any modicum of pain in labour, to the extent that the same agency is blurred and constrained within a particular, acceptable format of birthing 'right'. The wider structures of power that govern/ed these discourses need attention, for they diverge and converge in myriad ways. What Kitzinger termed 'technocratic birthing cultures' has had a long past, which included a long, tense and sometimes violent history of interactions between female midwives and wise women on the one hand and male obstetricians and healthcare professionals seeking to enter the birthing room on the other (c.f. Leavitt, 1986; Sandelowski, 1984). Structures of power embedded within patriarchy were at play here in and around the birthing room, where the protagonist, so to speak, was largely encouraged to lie back in silence.

In turn, in relation to the notion of the perinatal ideal that Chapter 2 constructed, these videos return us to the core ideology of neo-liberalism and the way in which the onus for change is placed on the individual. And indeed, far from these narratives being a question of representations alone of a specific style of natural birthing, different structures of power are at work here. These include access to hypnobirthing, and indeed the myriad options around fetal scanning (c.f. Stabile, 1992, on fetal imagery and maternal erasure), fetal and maternal merchandise, classes and postnatal options all require money, time (and presumably childcare for existing children, if any) to attend classes, to listen to tapes, to join online groups, and above all, these all require focus and commitment on the part of the individual – the mother. A large part of the unfolding literature within the hypnobirthing discourse and the infographics circulated online seem to develop problematic, nostalgic links (see also Dalmiya & Alcoff, 1993) between 'perfect' birthing practices in developing countries and obscuring critical issues surrounding childbirth and women in developing countries. These issues continue to include both problems around 'technocratic' birthing cultures in urban areas (c.f. Deyl, 2017) as well as high-risk neonatal and maternal situations in conditions of poverty (c.f. Bang et al., 2004), making birthing in developing countries far too complex to be exported unproblematically into the very Western, neo-liberal and largely middle-class practices of intensive motherhood (Hays, 1998).

Note

1 A version of this chapter has been previously published as Das, R. (2018b). Mediated subjectivities of the maternal: A critique of childbirth videos on YouTube. *The Communication Review, 21*(1), 66–84.

4 The two sides of support rhetoric[1]

The previous chapter considered the perinatal ideal as articulated in amateur home-birth *representations* of maternal sacrifice and transcending pain in the course of birthing. In this chapter, I move on from representations to considering articulations of the perinatal ideal in *talk* and discussion around birthing and labour. To do this, I bring together two small cases. The first is an analysis of 1930 posts from 12 discussion threads from an online parenting forum. The second presents a thematic analysis, following Riessman (2008), of themes arising from posts in a public Facebook group on hypnobirthing which includes a wide variety of practices before, at and shortly after birth, including relaxation, hypnosis, self-hypnosis and a steadfast rejection of medical intervention or even medical settings, to have a 'better' birth. Before I move on to the cases in question, I wished to address what it is that these cases – the forum and the specific variety of natural birthing group – represent and what my findings from these might and might not allow me to conclude in relation to the perinatal ideal. The parenting forum is an open forum with a subsection on childbirth and not specifically focused on any specific mode of birthing. The material on the broader forum is a popular site of analysis, and indeed, the childbirth forum itself might be analysed for myriad different purposes and frameworks. The Facebook group is focused very specifically on one particular style of natural birthing and sets out clear guidelines and rules on the specific discourses permitted, and these guidelines are maintained by group administrators and members largely, which I discuss later. In a way the Facebook group chosen is a somewhat 'niche' case study, because it focuses so clearly on a very particular style of birthing – hypnobirthing – which Chapter 3 focused on. While this focus on one particular niche is a valid approach in many ways, particularly so because it is an approach that is increasingly popular, what are the implications of such a selection in terms of what it tells us or does not tell us about broader maternal experiences on social media around birthing. This makes it imperative to consider what these particular forms of online content represent and what the scope of claims is that can be made from their analysis. I suggest that, at the very basic level, while the analysis applies to the cases I study primarily, the narratives invoked in them, around desirability of particular birthing styles, the complexity and nuance of these discourses of desirability having longer histories in agentic, critical, groundbreaking feminist midwifery movements, the subsequent moralising of birthing and wider perinatal responsibilities in conditions of the perinatal ideal and the arrival of new lines of exclusion and inclusion, speak not simply to the cases selected, but apply more broadly to the issues raised by scholarship I drew upon in discussing the perinatal ideal contemporary neo-liberal societies (c.f. Faircloth, 2013; Lee, 2008; Mack, 2016). So, my suggestion is not that hypnobirthing fora or one particular parenting forum represents all of contemporary discourse on birthing, but rather that these cases, one of which is a niche case, exemplifies wider debates, discourses and rhetoric that the perinatal ideal, as discussed in Chapter 2, has referred to. Also, as Hanson (2004) reminds us in her excellent account of the cultural history of pregnancy, pregnant bodies are always "viewed through constantly shifting interpretive frameworks" (p. 3), and as Longhurst remarks: "maternal bodies are socially, sexually, ethnically, class specific bodies that are mutable in terms of their cultural production" (p. 3). So, it is critical that we do not conceptualise pregnancy, birthing, motherhood and maternity as monoliths, and keep in mind that the material analysed here represents Western birthing and experiences of early motherhood in a Western country.

The cases

The Facebook group in question in this chapter is a very active group on a particular natural birthing technique. It had over 7,000 members at the time of analysis, including many birth-support practitioners such as doulas and hypnobirthing teachers, deriving most of its membership from mothers. The first step of the process involved a non-participant observation, many times a day, of discussions on the group for a year before analysis. Notes were made during this period, which were ethnographically motivated. After a year of observations, using NCapture – the Web material extraction tool on the qualitative analysis software NVivo – a dataset of all posts made on the group was generated, including the group moderator's opening post establishing the parameters of the group. The dataset automatically captured usernames of people who had made posts, the times of posts and all comments made in response to the posts. All posts were read and a purposive sample of posts was selected, the guiding criteria being that posts which were solely information-seeking were not considered. Instead, posts which spoke of experiences or which provided value-laden assessments of birthing options and choices and which asked for advice in terms of what action to take were considered in generating the purposive sample. All data was collected non-reactively. Non-reactive data collection focuses on data online in the public domain, and does not respond to, react or engage with participants online and lets phenomena unfold.

Whiteman's (2012) account of her work on publicly accessible bulletin boards discusses in detail the ethical considerations behind her decisions to not participate on the forums, to not seek informed consent and to acknowledge that not seeking informed consent and conducting analyses of publicly available data is not straightforward (Whiteman, 2012). The content posted on the forum analysed here are publicly available and do not require the group's membership to view content. One perspective on this material is that it might be treated as publicly available online material and be treated as such. But then, highlighting 'public' posts and recording them and giving them a degree of visibility greater than or different to what the posters might have anticipated counters such an argument, or at least strips it of the apparent ease with which it is often presented. This remains surrounded in nuance and complexity as conversations around ethics and public material demonstrate. As AOIR (2012) articulates "individual and cultural definitions and expectations of privacy are ambiguous, contested, and changing. People may operate in public spaces but maintain strong perceptions or expectations of privacy" (p. 6). As posters on Facebook are not anonymous and appear rather with their real names, all names were anonymised before analysis, although, in keeping with unfolding discussions of Internet research ethics, anonymity and pseudonymity are not the only ethical issues which might arise.

For the parenting forum, I conducted a thematic analysis, following Riessman (2008), of themes arising from 1930 posts in 12 discussion threads on a parenting website. This is a website known for a largely, if not solely, middle-class membership and for its tolerance of swearing, highly spirited and occasionally very heated arguments (Pedersen & Smithson, 2013). Although it is an online forum that anyone can sign up to and access, it is predominantly British and most posters are resident in the U.K. It started in 2000, and has since then grown into more than an online forum with very many topics and subtopics. It regularly supports and organises campaigns, lobbies on issues around women and children's well-being, frequently sees politicians, authors, journalists and other public figures make an appearance for scheduled web chats and its views are often sought in the print media. The forum is moderated around a system of Talk Guidelines and through a system of community reporting and central monitoring of reports, but individual posts are not vetted before they are posted.

A purposive sample of 12 threads ('threads' are the term for discrete topics of discussion) was selected after applying keywords such as 'birth stories', 'positive birth, 'birth trauma', 'negative birth' and 'labour stories' when searching the database of threads. The threads had diverse titles, ranging from ones specifically created for birth trauma support to those making it verbally clear that they solely wish to hear positive stories of labour. They are similar, in that nearly all of them were part of the 'childbirth' discussion topic and sought either help or information rather than simply posting to share one's own story. They are different in their diverging degrees of openness to positive and traumatic accounts. Discussions threads ranged between high traffic ones with more than 300 posts and low traffic ones with under 50 posts.

Riessman (2008) speaks of how "talk among speakers is interactively (dialogically) produced and performed as narrative" (p. 105). Riesmann's account of the nature and purposes of storytelling is particularly relevant for this project, where she says:

> storytelling is a relational activity that encourages others to listen, to share and to empathize. It is a collaborative practice and assumes that tellers and listeners/questioners interact in particular cultural milieus and historical contexts ... We ask why was the story told that way?
>
> (Riesman, 2013, p. 170)

Narratives for analysis are almost mainly long, detailed, autobiographical ones – like a single person's story or one single interview transcript. In an interesting essay, Georgakopoulou (2007) questions this, and reminds us of the importance to pay equal attention to what she calls 'small stories'. These, in her words are:

> a gamut of under-represented narrative activities, such as tellings of ongoing events, future or hypothetical events, shared (known) events, but also allusions to tellings, deferrals of tellings, and refusals to tell. These tellings are typically small when compared to the pages and pages of transcript of interview narratives. On a metaphorical level though, small stories is somewhat of an antidote formulation to a longstanding tradition of big stories .. the term locates a level and even an aesthetic for the identification and analysis of narrative: the smallness of talk, where fleeting moments of narrative orientation to the world (Hymes, 1996) can be easily missed out on.
>
> (p. 146)

At the beginning of the project, I wrote to the administrators of the website seeking consent from them to use material from their discussion boards for analysis and I was informed I could freely do so – the posts are not protected from public viewing or use (although my previous discussion of the muddiness of consensus on consent, privacy and ethics on 'public' material still apply here). All posters are pseudonymous on the forum, and should one wish, one might retrace a poster's posting history and begin to bring together a story that could potentially identify the person concerned ('outing' someone, in forum language), although the website allows a name change function. Keeping this in mind, I have not used pseudonymous forum names of posters.

A cathartic, rationalising and empowering space

On the online parenting forum Mumsnet, the hearing, telling, recounting and circulating of birth stories works within a critical circuit of interpretive devices which are simultaneously the products of interpretation (of others' stories) and the devices/lenses through which one's own births and others' births are interpreted, contrasted and even compared. One's own story is a part of this hermeneutic circuit (Gadamer, 2002), an experience which has been pre-mediated by the readily available range of stories one has heard before and expectations which have been established through a very wide range of resources.

Speaking about birth, after birth, outside of the clinical and time-limited contexts of debriefing serves as cathartic and therapeutic purposes for many women. One poster says: "This thread has made me cry, which I think I haven't done enough of". Another says: "I've never wrote it all down like that before and it's actually upset me all over again. It obviously just doesn't go away. This is kind of like therapy though". The sense of community, amity and solidarity that comes through on childbirth forums is striking, although, as the next section will evidence, this peer support often has other less convivial dimensions attached to it.

One poster says: "I may as well start with my story, it may help others to both open up and to be able to identify how their trauma will/may manifest itself". Responding to the stories that others tell becomes an act within this circuit which positions all interpretation and understanding as preceded and resourced by a background of pre-understanding that goes before these, including one's own judgements, and hence suggests that there cannot be an understanding that stands truly on its own (Gadamer, 2002). This circularity, between the present and its past suggests that "our truths are made possible by a shared background of life into which we are initiated, and into which we contribute, through our dialogues and interactions with others" (Martin, Sugarman & Thompson, 2001, p. 197).

It is important here that we pay attention to the nature of online discussion groups – they afford an immediacy to the exchange of stories, the scope for a range of interpretations, prejudices and understandings to co-exist on the same visual unit (the full screen), the scope for messages to be removed by forum administrators and be replaced by deletion messages and the very own language of emoticons, abbreviations and terminology specific to a particular forum. Storytelling on childbirth forums is discursively recognised and analysed by posters as useful for those that will lurk but not post, read but not share or those not pregnant yet. One poster reminds everyone of the importance of not just reading and expressing, but also of supporting and reaching out:

> There have been previous threads on which people have outpoured their experiences but acknowledgement and discussion is more than each of us telling our own experiences, so I ask that not only do we tell our own stories but we acknowledge other's and help them to discuss their past too.

Storytelling and listening to stories around childbirth becomes an important device through which women debate and disagree with institutions and structures, including medical systems, linguistic and discursive devices used socially in speaking about birth and of the systems within and against which women operate in birthing. One poster states categorically: "There are some problems I think in the language that is used around childbirth". There is a sense of protest which cannot be boxed into the tick boxes of complaint forms of medical institutions that becomes evident in the critique of discourse and language. One poster remarks:

> The language of midwifery is laden with unhelpful emotions I did not 'give birth' as I had an emergency c section after I 'failed to progress'. I previously have had a medical management of a miscarriage as I had 'retained products' and the doctor told me he would prescribe 'abortion pills'. Labels can be so unhelpful.

The Facebook natural birthing group, sitting close to the natural birthing movement, shows that a large part of the discourse on the group is about alternative and complementary practices, which lie outside of the periphery of Western medical institutional practices. The sharing of resources on positive affirmations, including visual displays such as charts and flashcards, reinforcing that a woman's body is her biggest resource in birthing, pictures that are overtly 'positive' in terms of sunrays filtering through the woods or the wide, open expanse of oceans and skies and the sharing of wisdom on non-medical practises, including aromatherapy, naturopathy and homeopathy, feature regularly and strongly in the group. Resource sharing, solidarity, distantiation from medical procedures and establishments and a strong sense of supporting each other features in these discussions. This involves a critique of both norms which are considered to be standard in medical institutions (e.g. the induction of labour) and words which are used in common parlance (e.g. pain, contractions, overdue etc.). This critique can be mapped on to the critique of technocratic, medicalised, obstetric cultures and serves as the site of friendship and solidarity, as is evident in this exchange below:

> My husband tells me not to criticise her (a midwife) as she's only trying to help. But I said "hey it's my birth I get to question and criticise anyone I want". Feeling defeat.
>
> Ilana
>
> Sadly midwives who tend to fall at the end of the medicalised birth spectrum can see birth plans as a nuisance. Stick to your guns.
>
> Melissa
>
> Please don't let her deviate you from the path you believe is best for you.
>
> Rihanna

There is vitality, cooperativeness and real agency in the support extended between mothers as they reject and oppose medical advice and technocratic labour cultures. These have remarkably positive and even empowering roles to play in the lives of women, who, for instance, like Charlotte, feel helpless and overwhelmed at the thought of labour and birth. There is a strong emphasis here, on women sticking with each other, in their united rejection of medical procedures and institutions.

These fora seemed to regularly open up a space for women to discuss the overpoweringly affective and profoundly difficult experiences of the materiality of birth trauma at a physical level. While online information about physical trauma is readily available, the emotional dynamics that accompany, for instance, the real, lived injuries of a forceps birth or the realities of requiring months of physiotherapy to cope with higher degree tearing following a vaginal birth are often topics mothers only felt able to discuss in the anonymity of the online. One mother who experiences a sense of delinking with her own body, presents her narrative as one of disconnection and a sense of not being present almost with one's own physical self:

> That's the other thing; ordinarily your 'bits' are your private property, but after a birth ... I felt totally alienated from that end of my body, like it wasn't mine any more, plus it was kind of rearranged.

The emotional role played by storytelling is significant. These spaces become areas where discussions of one's most private thoughts are (usually) acceptable, unless these thoughts venture into the ambivalent territories – such as the sharing of difficult or traumatic birth stories, which I move on to in the next section. A poster who has felt detached from her baby since birth is able to speak of difficult and often socially unacceptable emotions:

> My daughter doesn't feel like mine. She feels like a child I'm babysitting for or something. That was why I couldn't carry on breastfeeding – it felt wrong and it still feels wrong sometimes to change her bum.

This quote above makes sense when read against the ample literature on maternal ambivalence (Adams, 2014; Raphael-Leff, 2010), which grasps the complex, fluid and constantly morphing nature of motherhood, as thoughts such as the above may find little space and social acceptance. Madge and O'Connor note "the construction of mother as a category is not a pre-given, coherent and stable subject position" and maternal ambivalence such as the poster's above is an integral part of motherhood, "*the ambivalent holding together of love and hate*" (Adams, 2014, p. 10), and sometimes even a positive force (Raphael-Leff, 2010). As Raphael-Leff identifies, not being able to speak about ambivalence freely works as an exclusion which "compels mothers to hide conflictual and shameful feelings from professionals – and from themselves" (p. 1). Women post periodically, seeking examples and instances of these stories, as these are the stories that are most often sought.

One poster actively encourages others to share their concerns about birth: "I genuinely loved every minute of the labour and birth, and I'm no lentil weaver! Don't be scared, go with the flow. What's worrying you?" These accounts display most frequently narratives of conviviality, fellowship and solidarity. One poster reassures another:

> you're designed to give birth just like any other animal – and no other animal screams in pain when they are giving birth, it doesn't have to be like you see on TV. Being scared just makes you tense up then your muscles won't work effectively. Most women don't have a medicalised experience – you just tend to hear the horror stories and not the good ones.

A significant role of birth narratives is the sense of empowerment that is shared from one woman to another. The empowerment, which is voiced through the sharing of positive experiences, short labours, drug-free labours, active births and births at home, is a clear way in which women encourage each other to reject medical interventions, and indeed medical actors and establishments, in line with the philosophies of 'natural' birthing discussed previously. Equally, as an instance of camaraderie, but perhaps also indicating how moralised and heavy such topics have become in contemporary society, findings across my cases point to a significant amount of self-censure and management being taken on by mothers who have had positive experiences. Mothers expressing guilt at having an 'easier' time than others, indicating a subtle sense of competition and comparisons in birthing, mothers with positive experiences discursively demonstrating a stepping away from praise of any kind, mothers who have had difficult experiences positioning a positive experience as down to individual luck and a clear sense that traumatic experiences are often down to individual failings in some way.

Some of these discourses contradict each other; but that precisely is the nature of these discussions. Mothers often express a sense of guilt at having had an 'easier' time and do the interpretive work of reading other narratives to make sense of whether their own, personal, highly individual narrative can be classed as 'easy' or 'difficult'. As one poster says: "I actually had it pretty easy compared to some of you", or another: "I feel like a bit of a loon posting this on here because you ladies have all had it much worse than me". This links also to the verbally apparent stepping away from praise that is displayed by many posters who perceive themselves to have had an easier time. Both these posters and those who have had negative experiences class a 'good' birth as a function of individual good luck. One says: "If you're lucky enough to be able to cope with the pain with minimal pain relief, then good on you", while another remarks: "I hear 'you did really well' as a comment on the woman's incredibly good fortune, not a compliment on anything they actively achieved". Under this umbrella, one might also include substantial amounts of self-regulation in speaking about something that has become so laden with cultural attributes that the sharing of stories is no longer as simple as it might look:

> I think one of the reasons for the horror stories is that some people do have bad experiences so it can feel quite smug to be going on about your wonderful home births when you're not sure if the person/people you're speaking to has had a different birth.

Discursive and perceived silencing of 'horror stories'

A significant amount of emotional energy is invested in these discussions it seems into the mode, duration and type of birth and the degrees of pain relief involved. This energy is played out in discussions of birth online and is similar to Lee's account (2008) of infant feeding getting tied firmly into maternal identity work. The mode of birth and the use or rejection of pain relief become moralised indicators of ideal and less-than-ideal births, and therefore graded nuances emerge in terms of how 'well' a mother is perceived or perceives herself to have done in giving birth.

Discussions online, especially when people seek 'positive' birth stories, can display an aversion to traumatic or difficult stories being shared. The sharing of 'horror' stories is not something actively encouraged (there are separate threads created for trauma support) and a number of discursively apparent rhetorical strategies are evident in the silencing of difficult accounts. One of these is to paint the telling of a difficult story as a strategy, as one poster says: "When you are pregnant people always come out with the horror stories as they seem more interesting", or that "people definitely love to tell a gruesome story (or 12) to pregnant ladies". That a birth story needs to be 'interesting' and that the sharing of difficult experiences is a strategy to make it so ties in also with a general aversion to these stories.

This is displayed often as an attempt to avoid and avert – what has not been heard will do no harm. A poster says: "I remember telling everyone 'I don't want to know' before they started speaking if I knew where it was going". This is evident also in countless threads asking for solely positive accounts and actively discouraging the sharing of horror stories. The fact that a general discussion board needs to have separate support threads, clearly titled with birth trauma, for instance, shows that the space available to speak freely about childbirth difficulties or feelings of disappointment is limited. The rhetorical devices employed to close down convivial spaces for sharing difficult stories is sometimes more actively voiced. For example, one poster is told:

> It is ok for you to decide to have a C-section but starting a thread to try and alarm people into agreeing with you is not really that helpful is it? Please for goodness sakes do talk to someone about this so you can weigh up the risks and get it in proportion.

Difficult experiences are as varied as they can be, and yet rhetorically they are often grouped together, as though they were a homogenous mass that can eliminated and avoided in the run-up to a birth. This is a simplification of birthing experiences and accounts that becomes evident in comments which seek to enlist a very wide-ranging set of experiences into a single stream:

> It just seems like everyone has horror stories! And not just the people who are overly keen to share horrific stories – for all my family and friends who have had babies over the past few years its been a litany of forceps, 4-day labours, emcs, inductions with pain off the scale, filthy hospitals …!

Sharing 'negative' stories is not simply a question of sharing experiences after birth. The voicing of fears and anxiety is often bounced back to the individual in a way that preserves fears and concerns as the individual's responsibility alone:

> The only thing that leaps out at me is that you seem to be unsure about your choice and trying to justify it – regardless of whether you feel able to admit this to yourself or not. Perhaps this is due to personal doubts or due to the reaction you have had from others, but I don't think anyone but you can resolve this issue for yourself.

The sharing of 'horror' stories as a strategy, the grouping together of 'horror' stories into one homogenous narrative, the verbal shutting down of difficult accounts, the projection of fears as self-doubt or scaremongering are findings that align with the discursive silencing of negative accounts. It is noteworthy to mention that if people post seeking advice specifically for birth trauma, advice is often found from posters in the same boat. It is the more routine, everyday, even mundane discussions of birth and birthing that dominates online forums or even offline conversations as reported online, which involve this subtle silencing. This also links closely to the perceived silencing of difficult stories, which in the absence of an overt, immediate rhetorical silencing, as evident in the quotes above, nonetheless lead women to feel judged or silenced – as the example below will demonstrate. This perceived judgement is something that speaks significantly of the wide cultural attributes associated with natural and 'good' birthing rather than something that can be read at face value of an individual being oversensitive.

One poster writes about clinical evidence for natural birth thus: "absence of proof of harm is not proof of lack of harm … Infant formula is a commercial product. Surgical birth is a medical procedure. There is no harm in discussing the evidence underpinning the public debate about these things". On the surface, this seems like a factual statement and one made, apparently, without judging the choices or experiences of another. It triggers a very strong response in someone: "You are exactly the kind of mother

I was referring to. No wonder women feel judged". This corresponds also, of course, to a degree of resistance to such pressures, perceived or real, but more importantly ties in to a broader point about the heavy moralisation about all things perinatal – something I return to in Chapter 5 in greater depth. The 'kind of mother' interpreted here is because the poster interprets a statement of fact ('surgical birth is a medical procedure') as a loaded, meaningful statement of judgement, which then causes distress. Whether or not this statement of fact was intended to be loaded is impossible to decipher within the methodology of non-participant observation, but more crucially, the heightened emotions that read this statement as loaded and meaningful must be contextualised within a broader, societal narratives with and within which women make sense of their births.

Feeling judged without being judged and feeling judged while being judged may well be separated in terms of the rhetorical devices behind them, but wider socio-cultural contexts and cultural attributes associated with motherhood and mothering form the backdrop to these interactions. Feelings of failure, self-doubt and a sense of not achieving goals that are set to be aspired towards form part of this picture. A poster mentions that a specific natural birthing technique did not work for her: "it made me feel much worse, postnatally, because I had this sense of feeling like a failure to deal with as well as the recovery from an episiotomy and forceps". Or, as another poster remarks, representing perhaps, a form of discursive resistance:

> As for suggesting that mode of birth actually matters to babies – that's your personal belief, and there's a whole interweb full of people who claim the same, although there's from what I can see not much sound scientific evidence around this, but a lot of philosophical theorising and romanticising.

One might then connect, at a broader level, whether the dismissal of the evidence behind natural birthing by some as above, might be tied to the real, lived experiencing of a particular ideal, with very strong socio-cultural attributes linked to it, personal experiences of deviating from that ideal (through circumstance or choice) and then rejecting, discursively, any evidence behind what has become widely idealised. As one poster phrases this personal experience of deviating from an ideal: "I just feel like it could have been an amazing experience and I chickened out of it", and another whose use of the word 'artificial' is particularly poignant: "The fact that I gave birth artificially annoys me".

Rhetoric around labour

Both the Facebook natural birthing group and the YouTube hypnobirthing videos, discussed previously, seemed to build a version of an ideal birth through a range of visual and rhetorical practices, curating the perinatal ideal. I turn attention first to the natural birthing rhetoric on the Facebook group, in particular the importance it places on terminology and phrasing. In this group, the very terminology adopted in society and in hospitals and birth centres is an object of critique, for the words themselves are interpreted as the gradual dumbing down of women's agency. The group is clear at the outset in that all posts must be about the gentleness and joy of birthing. The word 'pain' is forbidden from use in the opening post by the moderator. The group moderator's words state this clearly: "Please use gentle language when you talk on here and refrain (sic) from posting references to 'pain' or 'hurt' would be very helpful". The rules of telling one's story and of framing one's narrative are set, gently yet firmly, in stone here. Scripts that will not conform to the abolishing of specific words will not be tolerated – a particularly difficult instance of this rule-bound and almost scripted nature of this discourse is given later in this chapter. A simple rule – of avoiding the language of pain or anything difficult or traumatic – enables the production of a group identity which is simultaneously inclusive (of those that conform) and exclusive (of those who do not).

John Thompson's exposition of the management of visibility and the struggle for recognition (1995) in everyday life, both intrinsically mediated, prove particularly useful to make sense of these processes of inclusion and exclusion – the struggle of narratives, one over the other in these mediated communicative contexts involves and establishes frames of reference which align to a very specific set of maternal subjectivities. A specific kind of birth and indeed, even gradations in the desirability of different kinds of natural birth produce birth as essentially a cultural object, creating instead of removing pressures off the shoulders of women, sitting at uncomfortable intersections with the achievements of the natural birthing movement which critically questioned the often problematic medical framing of childbirth as inherently risky and demanding clinical, hospital-based settings by default (see Hausman, 2005).

Maternal instinct is valued highly in the group. Mother's instinct appears to be inherently right and women are supported emphatically within the community to do their utmost best by their children by rejecting intervention, refraining from using certain words and by speaking of positive, joyful experiences. It is noteworthy that at heart, these very discourses quite rightly were central to the feminist midwifery movement, the successes of which are beyond dispute. But the valorisation of instinct in this setting, within broader norms of avoiding pain discourse is intriguing, for it erects new exclusions. The emphasis on maternal instinct is evident, below which resonate with Bamberg et al. (2007) theorisations of how narrative is made use of to present, produce, maintain and reproduce a coherent story to tell, which operates, in this case, within a particular and specific vision of maternal subjectivity – the joyful mother, enjoying a joyful pregnancy to give birth painlessly.

> Your instinct knows best. I have baby 2 due in May and if she shows up again, I might tell that midwife where to stick it! Believe you can xx.
>
> Kiera

> Please don't let her (the midwife) make you feel like you are not doing the best for your baby. Your baby is not born yet. Doing what is right for you is what is right for your baby because your health has such an impact on your child's right now.
>
> Clarissa

This emphasis on instinct runs clear and deep throughout and is grasped perfectly by Tyler and Baraitser's reminder of the intensely mediated nature of these discourses centring around the birthing mother as they observe: "if pregnancy was previously imagined as a passive, abject and ordinary physical state to be stoically borne in private, today pregnancy is a disciplinary 'body project' which women are instructed to covet and enjoy" (2013, p. 7). They grasp perfectly the pendulum shifts in our mediated frameworks of reference in speaking about birth and birthing bodies. On the one hand, this framework represents the core premise of natural birthing – a critical questioning of white-coated obstetrics and a return of what is natural. On the other hand, despite the emphasis in this discourse on maternal *choice*, there are boundaries and limits placed on what maternal behaviour will be supported, what will merely be tolerated and what is most unwelcome. The gentle reminder at the outset to not use words such as pain removes the first level of choice, for instance. Many women in the course of the fieldwork in the project this work emerges from noted that verbalising pain, including even swearing profusely in labour, gave pain a recognition, a legitimacy, and that helped them in recognising the hard work that labour truly is and that nothing is quite as extreme perhaps for the body. And yet, in placing strict guidelines on the terminology that is permitted and that which is not seems to turn a full circle – from a critique of obstetrics and a return to belief in one's own self (by rejecting the word 'pain') to a discursively visible silencing of women who must conform to the norms of the group and not speak of pain.

One of the key devices used in the group to filter out narratives that do not conform is the device of the 'trigger warning'. There is bravery and courage ascribed to not feeling or speaking of pain or suffering, and any accounts which do speak of pain or of women's choices in asking for or accepting pain management are filtered out or accepted with a 'trigger warning'. For instance, a moderator has edited a post that speaks of a difficult birth (if at all this is permitted to remain on the site) by saying: "Warning: May contain triggering material". The mother who has spoken of difficulty has created a narrative, told a story which has been discursively identified as a 'trigger'. Triggers are to be avoided and therefore, her story has already been mediated to be the other – in relation to whom the rest of the stories are to be read, normalised and accepted. One of the functions of the device of trigger warnings is unwritten blame and guilt – one has posted content which may trigger others. Blame and guilt both have key role to play in the intensive mothering discourse (see also Orgad & De Benedictis, 2015) with failing to perform according to these standards resulting in self-blame and guilt (Barnes & Power, 2015), and blame being placed on 'failing' mothers by the popular press and institutions. While trigger warnings aspire to protect, they become by default a policing of women's narratives about birth which allows certain narratives to be opened up and others to be closed down – mediating experiences selectively.

The mother not doing the 'right' thing or not doing well enough is of course sometimes visible only on probing. Birth stories which are celebrated seem to be the ones that involve no pain relief; a mother who battles through all possible odds in bearing pain whilst not calling it pain is the mother who shall feel no pain in labour. These stories receive the highest number of replies numerically and are posted in the group straight away. On the odd occasion a mother wishes to share her difficult experiences; however, this goes against the ethos of sharing only positivity and joy. An excellent example of the relative status ascribed to birth stories is below, which showed up during my yearlong observation of the group, and has since then been edited, including the editing out of certain comments by posters. In the instance below, two occurrences make the semantic status of difficult experiences clear. The gist of a woman's birth story is summarised in one, painful sentence: "I am currently in a rehab to walk because in all the maneuvers to get her out. I have muscle and nerve damage. It's not what I ever expected and I'm just so glad she's alive with us". This story however was unlike other stories – and not allowed to be posted on the group directly. Instead, the moderator made the original post using the word 'trigger', but the woman's story itself did not appear on the post. An edited, shortened version of the story was then posted in the comments. Immediately, a set of successive comments were posted in response to this powerful account of a woman's very real struggles, which involved abuse and chastising the woman for sharing negativity. Eventually, these comments were taken down. Overall, however, this story disappeared into the history of the group drawing only very few comments from posters – a stark contrast to the overwhelming, sometimes 10s or over a 100 comments in solidarity and support for 'positive' accounts. This works well with the architecture of social networking sites such as Facebook – the fewer comments something receives, the lower it slips in a news feed, and the lower it slips in a news feed, the longer it takes for a viewer/user to spot the story sliding down fast along a list of other stories generating more comments.

Under conditions of the perinatal ideal, this celebration of instinct, of the good mother doing her absolute best to give birth in a certain way, is framed as a rebuttal and rejection of hyper-medicalisation, but equally involves the establishment of a clear protocol for how to birth 'well', how to be responsible for understanding what qualifies as a 'good' birth and how that is the only route to a healthy baby. This framework is also part of a middle-class discourse that is complete with the attendance of often expensive classes, which requires rigorous practice and vast amounts of self-regulation to avoid thinking of pain in birthing. These communication practices, like all communication practices, may work to selectively silence and marginalise or highlight and bring to relief the voices and experiences of others. Through the sharing of stories on social media, the circulation of blogs, images, infographics, natural imagery and audio tapes, for each vision of 'good' births, there is created by default an image of birth that are not good enough. Births that are good births seem to have clearly established parameters and need to be worked towards intensively, methodically and with focus. A non-medical setting, no requirement of pain-relieving medication, no interventions, no noise, absolute calm and relaxation paints the picture of the ideal birth – and the ideal birthing woman who has done her job well – attended classes, practised affirmations, listened to self-hypnosis tapes, practised movements with her birth partner, consciously avoided any exposure to accounts of difficult births, walked away from any woman who seeks to speak of her difficult birth story. On the one hand, this is empowering for it is a rejection of fear, doubt, anxiety and an embracing of a natural process – a hard-fought outcome after many decades of silenced women in stirrups surrounded by white coats and intravenous drips. On the other hand, the articulation of this outcome into socially mediated codes of good birthing and the responsibilities that come with it establish new norms and new ideals to be aspired for.

One woman on the group epitomises this ideal by speaking of her 'nightmare' birth experience. In this narrative, one woman says:

> I was screaming from panic and pain. So loud that nurses were trying to hold me down. I ended up wanting an epidural, and when they attempted to give it to me it was unsuccessful. And then my baby was born in a scary, loud, chaos (sic) environment.

She is then reassured and directed by fellow posters to seek hypnotherapy to free herself of these fears. The epidural is a key protagonist in this nightmare. After the victories of establishing women's choice and agency in rejecting the passivity of women in labour (this victory still un-achieved around the world), a woman who actively chooses or wants any form of medical intervention, even if it is pain relief, in her own words, is poised to fail in her quest for a good birth, as she 'ended up' wanting an epidural. The words 'ended up' make it clear that, for her, needing or wanting support to cope with pain is an outcome of defeat and screaming (a normally comprehensible bodily response to physical pain that we otherwise allow for a variety of life situations) is not an acceptable response in labour. Labour and birth which involves screaming as a response to a natural yet extreme physical process or labour and birth which requires the numbing of pain is a story of nightmares. Indeed, as another woman demonstrates, if one has 'negative' stories (worries, bad experiences) to share and seek support for, the protocol is to not post on the group directly about it, but to warn others seeking avoidance of anything negative prior to posting. She posts: "Negative post so I will write in comments. But some advice welcomed!". These stories on social media are part of the hermeneutic circle within which childbirth is increasingly mediated. Like all processes and institutions of contemporary societies, birth and labour cannot now be thought of outside of the frameworks of mediation. Responding to others' stories circulating on Facebook, Twitter or parenting forums like BabyCentre or Mumsnet is one act within a circuit which shapes all future interpretations and understanding (Gadamer, 2002). This circularity, between the present and its past, suggests that "our truths are made possible by a shared background of life into which we are initiated, and into which we contribute, through our dialogues and interactions with others" (Martin, Sugarman, & Thompson, 2001, p. 197).

Part and parcel of preparing intensively for birth, under conditions of the perinatal ideal, is the active work that is demanded of women in preparation for birth, as I have identified above. This also includes the work involved in keeping everything except positivity at bay. This means that women who have had difficult experiences must not be listened to and only positive stories must be heard. As Natalia requests on her post: "any tips please xxx – PLEASE (capitalised in the original) only positive Notes/ideas rather than any negative experiences". These narratives underwrite discursive and rhetorical devices which actively close down discussions of births and experiences that have not fallen into the vision of the ideal birth and contribute to the formation of the maternal individual online as a neo-liberal subject, incorporating very middle-class values of self-control, expensive and rigorous preparations and classes. This links the present discussion on birthing and pregnancy online to wider discussions of neo-liberal discourses around good motherhood and good births and the work involved in mothering and childcare. In keeping with Lee's (2008) empirical work with the self-perception and identity of mothers who have had to or chosen to feed their babies infant formula, research with women who have aspired for, prepared but have not had what would be called ideal births or completely natural births, may reveal insights about mediated discourses at work in society, in the space that falls between the agentic, critical, rightful revival of women's bodies and voices against obstetric practice on the one hand and a pervasive discourse of intensive parenting in the face of anxiety and perceived risks on the other. Listening to women's voices on and offline as they speak about these experiences is the only way to begin to unpack that space.

Individualisation of birthing responsibilities

In discussing the perinatal ideal in Chapter 2, I spoke of it as a responsibilising and highly individualised ideology. As Lee notes (2008):

> It has been well established that mothering has, in modernity, been constructed as both the private responsibility of individual mothers,

> and also a matter of public scrutiny and intervention, with mothering practices defined as 'good' and 'bad' in expert and policy discourse (Lewis, 1980).
>
> (Lee, 2008, p. 468)

In reading women's interpretations of their own births and of images surrounding them in the context of an increasing move towards placing responsibility on the self and on individuals in contexts of the perinatal ideal (see also neo-liberal discourses on self-care), we can notice a shift away from the discourses of it taking an entire village to raise a child. In contrast to a wider recognition of the role of 'luck' in the process, many see to take on full responsibility of the experience on their own shoulders:

> My first birth was a horror story – but now I realise it was mainly because I tried to 'avoid' the birth- pretending it wasn't happening and then was too stoic when I should have been demanding. It meant I had all the wrong kind of intervention.

This individualisation of responsibility is evident in pregnancy advice, as has been studied by scholars (c.f. Lee, 2008), and manifests itself not just in terms of women making sense of hard times, but also in women's preparations for an aspired-for positive birth experience. One poster advises another: "Anyone can always try to treat you like a cretin, the difference is how you let it impact on you. Giving birth is a case of mindset – go in with a open one!" – words simultaneously empowering and individualising the tasks and responsibilities of giving birth. What is at stake in this individualisation of responsibility, risk perceptions and management and of dealing with outcomes? Critiques of individualisation (Beck, 1992; Beck et al, 1994) beckon an argument for a more collaborative, connected and diffused approach to birthing responsibilities, as opposed to the deeply fragmented individually invested mode. As these accounts show, these two narratives are often overtly visible in discourse. This is not always so, however. Even when the mode of birth as an indicator is stripped in discourse of its moralised baggage, women with varied experiences of birthing show discursive strategies of still working around these indicators in their narratives and interactions. This happens through either distancing themselves from a sense of achievement (when they fit in with what is perceived to be more laudable birthing choices and experiences) or perceiving themselves to have failed even when there is nobody who has told them so. The former subtly recognises that birthing naturally has medically and culturally ascribed authority and preference and therefore can alienate those who did not or could not fit in, thus displaying self-deprecating techniques, including humour, to not claim praise. The second, aware of these same culturally heavy indicators of 'good' births, displays a sense of having failed and going unrecognised even in cases where these attitudes have not been verbally, literally articulated to them.

So we see two cross-cutting discourses, blurring issues of agency, control and power, have emerged with regard to the now heavily mediated birthing body – a finding which applies to the visual logics of mediated hypnobirthing explored in Chapter 3 as well. However, historically, powerful, feminist agency located within and through the emancipatory feminist revival of women asserting themselves against the white-coated, often male, medical community, harking back to the introduction of the natural birthing movement in the U.S.A. and U.K. (Gaskin, 2003; Kitzinger, 2012b) foregrounded the critical importance of women's voices in the labour room. The more recent neo-liberal, self-regulating, self-managing, highly individualised discourse of ideal births and ideal birthing modes which sit within the perinatal ideal swings the pendulum, it seems, so far as to constrain that very agency. While medicalised discourses encouraging cultures of fear and anxiety around birthing typically remove women's control, many natural birthing discourses emphasise women's control and indeed, near-mythical victory over any modicum of pain in labour, to the extent that the same agency is blurred and constrained within a particular, acceptable format of birthing 'right'. The wider structures of power that govern/ed these discourses need attention, for they diverge and converge in myriad ways.

Conclusions

This chapter has contributed to a developing body of empirical work on childbirth and social media, by listening to women's talk online, how it frames discourses of birthing and how such talks worth within and feeds into the perinatal ideal. It has drawn attention to the contradictions, tensions and juxtaposition of contrasting discourses surrounding the birthing body, locating these within the perinatal ideal and its neo-liberal preoccupation with individualised, intensive maternity (c.f. Douglas & Michaels, 2005; O'Brien Hallstein, 2011). This chapter has complemented the empirical literature available around visual cultures of childbirth by exploring discursive cultures on these forums to show how they become a site where childbirth reveals itself as a baggage-laden subject of intensive motherhood of two contrasting sets of voices – one empowering and the other disempowering – with both seeming to represent historical shifts in attitudes to women, women's bodies and childbirth as a biological, social and cultural practice.

Crucially, these voices do not belong to two neatly divided camps, but are really best thought of as two sides of one coin, embedding one within the other. On the one hand, these platforms witness a welcome assertion of the knowledge that birth isn't something to fear, and that obstetricians and surgeons aren't necessarily the best birth attendants and that one should be confident about one's own body to take care of a natural process in the safe environment of the U.K. This is evidenced by many mothers sharing enabling, empowering stories with first-time mothers and aligns closely with the feminist revival of women-led, midwife-supported care for birthing women, which made a real statement against the white-coated, clinical obstetrics-led model where many women in the U.K., even a few decades ago, were asked (often by male doctors) to lie down and get on with it. The other side of this conversation, visible less frequently and perhaps more dramatically, on these forums is the muting of 'horror stories'. The first discourse has been historically monumental for women, women's agency and bodily autonomy, as indicated previously in this chapter. It has rescued women from being the passive recipients of a clinical and sometimes surgical process towards being active participants in birth. But the second discourse, as many mothers described, mothers whose 'horror stories' had been muted collectively, online and offline, represents the pendulum swinging the other way.

As Orgad remarks about the argument of scholars in feminist internet studies and development (2005):

> for them the significance and impact of online communication can and must be evaluated only in light of its actual consequences for the material conditions and cultural practices within which it is embedded. The fact that women talk to each other online, and that in this process peripheral matters gain public recognition, is not sufficient on its own. (p. 144)

Flipping Orgad's question about these sorts of online arenas in terms of whether they can "constitute more than anonymous therapeutic spaces" (p. 157) to inquire into their real, lived, positive potentials, one might ask the opposite question in the context of these sorts of parenting forums – can the hurt and guilt that one might walk away with from these discussions contribute to offline implications for women? Peer-to-peer support networks online are rapidly becoming popular, 24/7 avenues of wisdom sharing, virtual hand-holding and occasionally less positive platforms where those responsible for very young children, while feeling frayed, confused and exhausted, seek help. These platforms aren't to be dismissed as the general chatter of the networked world, not just for their potentials and possibilities in the face of public funding cuts, but because of the ways in which these conversations mirror and even shape the ways in which we, as a society, think and speak about children, parents and families.

Note

1 Versions of this chapter have been previously published as Das, R. (2017b). Speaking about birth: Visible and silenced narratives in online discussions of childbirth. *Social Media + Society, 3*(4). doi:10.1177/2056305117735753; and Das, R. (2017a). The mediation of childbirth: "Joyful" birthing and strategies of silencing on a Facebook discussion group. *European Journal of Cultural Studies*. doi:10.1177/1367549417722094.

5 Short-lived ties, lasting implications[1]

Up till now, this book has considered a few discrete sites where the perinatal ideal, as an individualising, moralising and responsibilising ideology, finds its way into and in turn feeds out of talk and representations. In doing this, my task has been to treat these sites as illustrative examples of the ways in which meanings around the perinatal circulate, are curated and sustain both inclusions and exclusions in relation to the perinatal in mediated, digital societies. In this chapter, I begin to look into these issues in the context of my fieldwork, where the focus shifts from discrete sites towards mothers' connections with each other and with their wider communities in the perinatal period. As this chapter presents findings on mediated, maternal interpersonal connections in the period before and immediately after childbirth, I consider the weight added to all topics to do with the perinatal from pregnancy to returning to work. In doing so, I focus on the role played by these often, although not always, short-lived social ties developed during this period and advance the central argument that digitally mediated interpersonal connections are critical components of contemporary motherhoods, but that these ties have complex positive and less than positive nuances in the perinatal period. Unpacking this argument in three steps, I first discuss how the moral weight of motherhood in neo-liberal societies, rendered particularly visible in the perinatal period, complicates a central boundary in the study of online interpersonal relationships between information and communication. Second, I note the relative significance, in emotional terms, of temporally contained social ties in digitally mediated perinatal connections. Third, I consider how the material and emotional roles of traditionally held-to-be-important offline maternal support networks are renegotiated, repositioned and even bypassed through online ties.

In the current context of austerity in the U.K., National Health Service (NHS) support for meeting mothers' needs in this regard, through face-to-face and regularly accessible interventions, has come under significant pressure, resulting in unmet needs (DoH, 2011). Simultaneously, with the burgeoning of a range of digital interfaces and sites, mothers have been seeking advice, support and fellow feeling online (c.f. Cheresheva, 2015; Gray, 2013; O'Connor & Madge, 2004; Pettigrew et al., 2016), although, as Chapter 7 elucidates, there is vast unevenness in contexts of use, access and practices. For those going online, these practices themselves can be located against now established practices of patients, vulnerable groups, stigmatised groups and parents going online for information and support (c.f. Amichai-Hamburger et al., 2013). However, there is as yet little analysis of these practices in a perinatal context, particularly in relation to the digital mediation of women's interpersonal connections, and the significance, including potentials and pitfalls, of these practices for the NHS and its current gaps in care for perinatal well-being. My analysis of online maternal discourse around childbirth in chapters 3 and 4, for instance, evidenced a complex juxtaposition of both supportive and exclusionary rhetoric, leading to mixed rather than uniformly inclusive or useful experiences for women online. There is evidence in favour of strong social connections and social support, encompassing instrumental, informational and emotional support for women perinatally (c.f. Leahy-Warren et al., 2011), in the context of this support itself being increasingly digitally mediated, as mothers go online on a variety of platforms. But we know little about the nature of ties, connections and relationships that result both online and offline (as a consequence of digital shaping), and the significance these hold for an understanding of digital sites in the perinatal months and in turn, for the ways in which the perinatal ideal is mediated. I draw upon this discussion to bring to relief that when these ties produce exclusions and reinforce divisions, they emerge out, produce and maintain possibilities of a maternal blame discourse, characterised by high amounts of maternal shame and mother blame, through the valorisation of individual, intensive and always gendered maternal narratives of sacrifice. However, they can also become sites of amity and solidarity which produce new inclusions and help fill gaps in pre-existing offline networks.

The normative and regulatory texture of *information*

As women increasingly go online to find information on both health issues and parenting (Bernhardt & Felter, 2004; Madge & O'Connor, 2006; Warner & Procaccino, 2004), one of the key findings from sociological scholarship on the Internet and interpersonal connections has been a perceived duality between information (and its seeking and provision) and communication (for emotional support, for instance). As Valkenburg et al. (2006) posit, feedback on the self and peer involvement – linked themselves to self-esteem and well-being – are more likely to happen during online *communication* than during online *information* seeking and provision. An example of information seeking for information alone is probably the case with Jemima. Jemima has three children, her eldest being nearly 18 when we spoke, and with a very big gap between her first and second. Her first birth was an unplanned pregnancy she went through at 16, where she haemorrhaged very badly, and then for her last birth she had pre-eclampsia and an emergency delivery where her tiny baby was born before she could find medical assistance, and the baby weight under four pounds at birth. When we spoke, Jemima had a distant and somewhat jaded approach to perinatality, speaking to me about her experiences in an almost detached manner. She speaks of information found online in a distant, detached fashion:

> I think I've gone onto like Net Mums and stuff a couple of times. Like when I was pregnant and just to find some answers to things like if I had a little worry in my head or ... You know? You always find them when you're pregnant, like how many times ... How much you're meant to feel the baby move ... and all that kind of stuff. So ... I would look online, kind of what the answer is.

Many in Jemima's position look for information online as information alone, so to speak, where such information does not apparently carry any affective or moral coding. But the vast majority of mothers provided and interpreted information as embedded within a variety of normative structures, and almost always loaded with value of one kind or another. Sometimes, as many of the examples which follow demonstrate, information might sit within regulatory structures of the perinatal ideal. At times, as evident from conversations with some migrant mothers, it might speak to other, equally gendered, normative structures in cultures of origin. So the normative and regulatory weighting of information which I speak of in this section might come from different, overlapping sources, whether part of the perinatal ideal as located within the intensive mothering discourse or not. Information about the perinatal manifests itself in a range of garbs, as discussed here, and all of it morally weighted and hence interpreted through weighted lenses. This applies not simply to perinatality potentially, but more widely to emotive issues with complex politics around them – for instance, parenting in later years or other health and well-being issues.

In this section, I pay attention to this difference that runs through the conceptualisation of digitally mediated interpersonal relationships, particularly in relation to parenting and motherhood, arguing that the *moral weight* of motherhood in conditions of the perinatal ideal, emerging from within the logic of intensive mothering and rendered particularly visible in specificities of the perinatal period (especially to do with issues such as birthing, breastfeeding, weaning and infant sleep), complicates these boundaries between information and communication. This means also that we conceptualise information itself as complex, graded, nuanced, formal and informal. While an obvious kind of information might, for instance, be a leaflet from a health organisation, an infographic produced on an informal natural birthing Facebook group, by either an informal advisor or a Doula, a variety of other things might also be classed or perceived as information, as might be information provided in interactive exchanges.

Runia is a second-generation migrant mother from Leicester. She experienced the perinatal period as what she described as a "cataclysmic incident, like some kind of an earthshattering thing", where she felt let down by overlapping circuits of support. At birth, she felt her partner and her mother did not quite believe the degree of pain she was in, as her partner appeared to her to be doubting the levels of her labour pain, and as her mother seemed to have forgotten labour altogether and kept saying that her own births were far easier. This was followed by her feeling stripped of choice in the hospital where she begged for pain relief and was denied it. In the early postnatal days, her son had an acute viral infection and had to be hospitalised, and she came under high amounts of familial pressure to formula feed and high amounts of healthcare professional pressure to breastfeed, and she felt torn and traumatised throughout her perinatal period. She expresses such a lack of choice as "you just listen to whatever they say, don't you. But maybe I didn't really research into it enough myself, but if I'd known more or said help me more ...". As she located the responsibility for things going wrong on her own shoulders, for not researching more or asking for help more rather than a broader system of pressures which did not support her, she turned to the world of peer-to-peer forums online to be able to make decisions for herself. But as she did so, all information she found sat within moralised, divided camps and contrasting and highly emotional networks of debate.

> It's not overly scientific.. it's just people's worries and then the information given is probably what everybody think is all different. You're like, so is that right or is that right ... or you look for another source to try and figure it out.

Runia speaks about how she commuted from one source of information online on Netmums and Mumsnet to another, till she, in her own words, found the 'right' information. In the context of real and perceived cultural pressures, both to exclusively breastfeed (which she was struggling to establish) on the one hand and to move to formula to increase baby's weight on the other (which she struggled to commit to), she spoke of finding the right information finally, which turned out to be a version of combination feeding. Information gathered till that point had felt restrictive and 'wrong' to her, something she described as 'not scientific'. Runia did extensive online searches for, encountered and interpreted a wide range and sources of information ranging from official leaflets as online PDFs to lay yet professional-looking infographics produced on online groups within the cultural paradigms and the associated moral weight attached to infant feeding methods (c.f. Lee, 2008).

Heeya is a secondary school teacher – a job she says she finds utterly rewarding – and was on maternity leave with an infant when we spoke. Heeya wanted to return to her job which she had loved for 11 years, but circumstances and practicalities around a new baby and a partner who would not take on primary care given his work conditions meant that Heeya was having to contemplate giving up her career. What complicated Heeya's situation further was that her baby was the outcome of rounds of infertility treatment processes, which meant that she needed to find additional sources of information and support through the assisted conception process, for which she turned to a range of different online platforms. She discovered very quickly that all information about the IVF process came with opinions which sat within people's own histories and practices and which generated simultaneous networks of inclusion and exclusion:

> I was on like Fertility Friends which, you know, during the IVF process and then while I was pregnant. That was really like a positive support network. Like compared to Facebook like ... There's a Facebook group, Babies Babies Babies that I'm part of. Sometimes there seems to be ... People tend to like be a bit more, not negative, but have their own sort of strong opinions and a bit like can be, not nasty, but just not very supportive sometimes when you need some information.

Niche groups, Heeya found, were more useful, where a degree of preselection had already happened and a degree of harmony and homogeneity established, for instance, on infertility treatment networks. Information she found on wider, more public forums, for instance, on Facebook, was often submerged in heavy, emotionally fraught debates on the simplest of queries and responses to these. Following Andreassen's (2017) findings on the normative and regulatory function of online intimacies, I posit that the morally laden nature of the perinatal complicates 'information', whereby information itself either contains or is perceived to contain a normative and regulative function. I note here that my argument applies both to one-way forms of information gathering, for instance, through the information collected from a leaflet, as well as information sought and provided through interactive interpersonal or community exchanges.

Glenda had six children and was happily building what she and her partner wanted – a large family. She had a perfect experience with her latest birth – it had been a calm water birth, the baby was healthy, they felt unrushed at the birth centre, could spend time together as a family and experienced it all to be 'lovely'. Feeding, however, did not quite work to plan, and she struggled to find information on feeding positions, encountering complex and conflicting information about it online across a range of peer groups. She sensed quickly whilst trawling through discussions for feeding positions and feeding routines that there was a:

> great pressure on mums to be the perfect mum, have the perfect birth, to have the perfect child that, you know, is only breastfed, doesn't have dummies. You know, you mustn't rock your baby to sleep. They might get used to it. You mustn't do this. I'm failing. You're failing from the offset.

Glenda, who herself struggled to establish and, in her own words, 'succeed' at breastfeeding, illustrated this, recollecting when she went online for information on infant feeding. Her response to the information draws in and speaks out of a range of established evidence and normative pressures the response to the information, being emotional, in the end:

> Everywhere I looked, the literature said breast is best. I felt so insecure and powerless. I think Netmums and Mumsnet are there to support mums, but they can be so cliquey. You have to be careful what you post there. You can feel quite insecure. It's very hard to gauge someone's feelings by what they're writing, the same as a text message. There's no emotion.

Glenda illustrates this, recollecting when she went online for information on infant feeding. Her response to information draws in and speaks out on a range of established evidence and normative pressures, the response to the information being emotional in the end. But Glenda was not alone in this. Reading information provided online about the hours taken during a short and relatively easy labour in a context of information being sought about duration of labour, for instance, proved to be triggering for a mother who had been left with traumatic injuries after birth. Likewise, I often found, when discussing infant feeding choices, information about the biological composition of breastmilk – conveyed through the words 'breastmilk contains antibodies tailored for the infant' – carried an affective weight, for it was interpreted through the pervasive societal lens of *breast is best* and the extended feeling reported among many formula-feeding mothers of guilt and shame (c.f. Faircloth, 2013; Lee, 2008) as a consequence of not breastfeeding.

As I discussed in relation to the perinatal ideal in Chapter 2 and the imperative to birth naturally, entirely free of medical interventions (c.f. Das, 2017; Mack, 2016) or the imperative to breastfeed exclusively and the intense relationship between maternal sense of self and identity in terms of the method of feeding (c.f. Faircloth, 2017; Lee, 2008), the many overlapping practices around weaning (c.f. Hanser & Li, 2017) and a variety of other perinatal issues relate to the new momism (Douglas & Michaels, 2005) under conditions of intensive mothering (Hays, 1998) where maternal sacrifice, and inseparability from the infant to do the 'right' thing for the infant, is posited to be the most natural choice, fitting into images of good mothering. I found in my fieldwork – information – even when presented as facts or statistics was almost always interpreted as carrying deeply normative parameters attached to it. This spanned official information, gathered from reputable online sources such as the NHS website or the NCT website or information read on online forums. Rather than these discussions presenting as outright disagreements online or even offline, mothers revealed through talk that they left online encounters of reading official as well as unofficial information, even when factually correct, feeling overwhelmed and burdened. This sense of burden, arising within the gendered, political and cultural logics of the perinatal ideal, renders itself particularly visible during the perinatal period and in turn, links the seeking and interpretation of information in information seeking encounters to deeply affective and physically sensate experiences of emotion for many mothers. This perceived and real weightiness of discourse, often presented as information, and its links to well-being is recognised by many mothers. As one mother said:

> I read in many places that normal childbirth this, or normal childbirth that. And then I myself never managed ... there was nothing normal about what happened with me. So – what was it then? Not normal? I felt like a massive failure.

Charmaine is originally from Portugal and moved to the U.K. recently, where she was completing a PhD, doing some teaching on the side and had a small baby when she spoke. She had a supportive partner but none of her own family around her and had experienced various perinatal difficulties, including a traumatic birth which had not gone according to plan. She spoke at length to me about her experiences providing information to someone who asked what labour is like, sharing openly the fact that she felt pain during labour – while sharing her birth story online. She was taken aback at the emotions it generated in a natural birthing community that operates rules against sharing information containing any mention of 'pain'. She says:

> If you're going to tell your story on hypnobirthing groups on Facebook, you will get deleted. You know, your story will get eliminated to a certain extent. When I finally ... did, I did say I'm going to use the word pain, because that's what I experienced, and as a human being, you know ... I had people coming and saying, you know, are you sure it was pain ... It's just the way you perceive it.

Charmaine talks about her experiences providing information to someone who asked what labour is like and sharing openly the fact that she felt pain during labour – while sharing her birth story online. She is taken aback at the emotions it generates in a natural birthing community which operates rules against sharing information containing any mention of 'pain'. Information sought perinatally is often affectively weighted, both by seeker and provider, and as my findings show, information carries emotional weight in this context and brings affective trails with it, blurring the lines, in perinatal relationships between information seeking and emotive, affective, communicative outcomes resulting as a consequence. My findings suggest that a clear separation between information seeking/finding and communication for emotional support is not entirely tenable in this context, owing to the morally weighted nature of the perinatal period. All women I spoke to, who mentioned seeking online information about infant feeding, childbirth, infant sleep or weaning, brought up emotive memories of both seeking information by actively reaching out to others online and responding to information they either stumbled across or received in response to active seeking.

Temporally inexpensive, affectively expensive

As Haythornthwaite (2002) notes, strong ties are usually long-term, voluntary, reciprocal, emotionally supportive forms of contact and lie at the heart of what Putnam (2000) called 'bonding capital'. Baym notes that weak ties are usually facilitated by digital media connections, while, in comparison, "resources exchanged in strong tie relationships run deep and may be emotionally and temporally expensive" (2015, p. 125). In what follows, I pay close attention to this characteristic of strong ties – the temporal and emotional depth – which is found to be unusual for the weak ties developed in much of digitally mediated interpersonal connections.

Violetta worked for the NHS in the middle of England and spoke to me about the risks of miscarriage and stillbirth logically and factually, herself being a professional in the healthcare sector. But while she spoke of a supportive and close bond with her mother, it emerged that it is within that supportive and close mother-daughter relationship that seeds of an idea that her body might reject her fetuses had emerged, particularly the more she aged, although she was in her early 30s when we spoke. She went on to have a traumatic first birth, which then led her to move to online and offline hypnobirthing courses to try to have a 'better birth' for her second time, intent on giving her second child a 'better start'. Violetta, below, says the following while speaking to me about her online interactions with a natural birthing adviser and practitioner, looking back at her perinatal months with her second child:

> I was gutted. I said to her … I said I'd really reconsider you using that video because as having gone through my first labour not being prepared, having two shots of pethidine and finally a spinal block, to now think back … I felt a failure as it was, but then to have that stereotype reinforced by someone describing someone as having a drugged-up baby just made me just feel awful … You feel like a failure and you don't feel like you're doing it the proper way or the natural way or as God intended or nature intended and stuff, and you do … It does make you kind of wonder, you know … Oh, maybe I wasn't strong enough or maybe I got coaxed into it or …

What the transcripts do not reveal is her visible, affective response to the memories of both her interactions with the practitioner and the audiovisual material presented as information on the right kind of births that she was given. On the one hand, the quote illustrates a previous point I made about the complex nature of information – and its seeking and provision – in all issues relating to the perinatal. On the other hand, I draw attention to the lasting strength and affective power, so to speak, of a temporally contained tie in the perinatal year that she looks back on – interactions and emotions which have permanently, it would seem, coded her own birth experience to her, such coding produced and maintained within a wider circuitry of representations and meanings and inclusions and exclusions around the perinatal that my discussions of the perinatal ideal in Chapter 2 has alluded to. This point – about the affective, and lasting strength of temporally contained yet emotionally expensive ties – became particularly evident in fieldwork with mothers looking back at the perinatal period, and recollecting their experiences of physical and social aspects of the perinatal (breastfeeding, post-birth difficulties), recounting a variety of digitally mediated weak ties, which seemed to hold, even months or years down the line, profound and transformative emotional significance.

Ties, of course, are often in flux in terms of levels of strength. Baym (2015) suggests that one of the processes through which weak ties morph into strong ties is self-disclosure, evidenced also in the literature on mediated intimacies (Chambers, 2013). My findings indicated throughout that self-disclosure on online connections are important and prevalent for perinatal mothers, and particularly critical for those experiencing depression and anxiety and finding it difficult to leave the house (c.f. Brunet & Schmidt, 2007; Valkenburg & Peter, 2007). Layla's perinatal journey was a particularly perilous one. She was diagnosed with sciatica and spent most of her pregnancy on crutches and could not walk properly. In addition, she and her partner both had fertility difficulties and their baby was a result of complex IVF treatment. This, she says, made her feel like she had failed, "because *it's the one thing a woman is supposed to be able to do, and I couldn't do it. And it made me angry, seeing other people getting pregnant like that and it did really make me emotional*". The birth was difficult, she could not move properly owing to her stitches. She was entirely incapacitated, her baby hospitalised and she could barely eat. She started feeling very low and her relationship with her partner deteriorated significantly, including at the time of our interview. To make matters even worse, her mother suffered a stroke a fortnight after she gave birth and passed away before her baby was six months old:

> You see on Facebook, people, oh, mum, baby doing well and everything. I think, I never had that. I am part of Mumsnet. You get a few nasty women on there that are a bit contradictive and a bit judgemental. They do get quite heated, quite nasty. Oh, God some of the women are quite nasty some of the things they say … I didn't bother talking to anybody, because I always got the phrase, you're pregnant. You're not dying. So it was just, okay, then, fine, don't waste my time.
>
> Layla

For Layla, amidst her desperation and isolation offline, online groups held the promise and potential for affectively significant ties. She did establish ties, albeit very short-lived ones. But they quickly taught her to not disclose, not establish intimacies, not expose herself and her struggles too much. Later, with a nearly two-year-old child with her, as she spoke to me, she spoke of these interactions, very often with tears in her eyes, excusing herself for doing so, gesturing to me often to turn off the audio recorder as we spoke about forum interactions. Two years on, then, from the very intense and early of the hazy days of the perinatal, short-lived mediated ties were still significant to her and coded much of the perinatal for her. The lines between weak and strong ties appeared to be more blurred in terms of perinatal interpersonal connections than one might expect, if not temporally, then emotionally. An account, this time of a positive and supportive but still temporally contained online social tie is provided here, when Marie speaks of her connections with a fellow mother on a forum supporting mothers of babies with colic:

> That's what I was doing, reading more of their stories, because I'm that sort of person that doesn't people feeling sorry ... I don't want people feeling sorry for me, because it will make me cry and everything. I like to be stronger and sharing that kind of problem, to me, would have made me a bit weaker. But that's how I felt, anyway, it would make me so emotional, which is not what I wanted to be.
>
> Marie

Marie recollects the comfort, solidarity and support she found in the connection with fondness as she thinks back, but confesses to never disclosing her own experiences – not through a sense of protecting her privacy or not being comfortable enough to self-disclose, but because she found it too emotionally difficult to let the other person reach out and feel for her.

Putnam's (2000) draws out the distinction between bridging and bonding social capital that relies on what sociological scholarship on online ties has theorised as weak ties: "connections between individuals who may provide useful information or new perspectives for one another but typically not emotional support" (Granovetter, 1973; Ellison et al., 2007, p. 1146). Putnam posits that homogenous ties of solidarity between 'people like us' result in less social inclusion, whereas weaker ties of loosely connected people might do the reverse (see Edwards, 2004). But these emerge to be complex in terms of perinatality. On the one hand, this period is indeed marked by the seeking and establishment of many short-lived, loosely connected, digitally mediated social ties between individuals and groups which may not know each other or may rarely meet face to face. However, while the vast majority of the digitally mediated social ties mothers establish during the perinatal period are short-lived, these are not necessarily emotionally or temporally inexpensive – and can come with heavy stakes and costs attached, generate significant inclusions and exclusions and seem to have apparent shaping roles in terms of offline stronger ties.

This draws attention to their immediate, temporal significance from perinatal well-being perspectives. In order to fully grasp the consequences of these ties for maternal well-being, it is critical that both the momentary and lasting impacts of these ties are investigated. As instances presented in this chapter demonstrate, the lines between a weak tie providing 'useful information' and becoming a momentary but nonetheless critical emotional support (or source of distress) are more blurred than straightforward. The inclusivity and exclusivity arising out of these short-lived mediated ties are more nuanced than straightforward.

In this context, I turn attention now to mothers' mediated self-disclosure of perinatal difficulties and the complexities around openness, anonymity and pseudonymity in the process. Evidence shows that online interfaces might often facilitate self-disclosure, particularly for those finding it difficult to access or open up in face-to-face settings (Brunet & Schmidt, 2007; Valkenburg & Peter, 2007). Two points about the role of self-disclosure in relation to online social ties beg reflection in the context of perinatality. First, both on Facebook groups dedicated to specific aspects of perinatality and on tweets relating to postnatal depression (bearing hashtags such as #pnd, #maternalmentalhealth etc.) and in the course of fieldwork, it became clear that communicating information about perinatal well-being issues comes hand in hand with the affective disclosure of individual experiences, often communicated through a series of tweets or through hyperlinks to individual blogs or websites. This is in keeping with Chambers' (2013) findings, which suggest that "self-disclosure has ... become the engine that drives new relationships" (pp. 46–47). The second aspect about perinatal self-disclosure in online ties is its simultaneous public-private articulation. Twitter data is public, usually, and this also demonstrates amidst users of this hashtag an acceptance of the simultaneously public and private nature of emotional self-disclosure. This is clearest in the microblogging activities of mothers acting on Twitter as awareness raisers, either operating on their own or as part of small third sector charities and community support organisations. Certain user profiles on Twitter, maintained by mothers who have undergone or are experiencing postnatal depression and anxiety and developing awareness raising campaigns (such as #pndchat or #babylosshour on Twitter), make use of public self-disclosure to build interpersonal affective connections that are mobilised in the circulation of information – from self-help advice to alerting people about formal support channels to petitions and activism. An instance, here from a mother who suffered from postnatal depression and is now an awareness raiser and host/participant on the regular #pndchat Twitter discussion elucidates this:

> As someone who has been through the darkness of postnatal depression with the fear that the sun will never shine again; it will. There is hope and help out there, please take that super brave step to seeking help. You are not alone.
>
> (#pndhour)

This tweet, disclosing her own struggles are part of a series of tweets communicating awareness raising information, information about signs and symptoms of postnatal depression, avenues for help etc. Likewise, interview transcripts revealed to me time and again that morally heavy and affectively weighted issues of the perinatal, around birthing, feeding, sleeping or weaning, always brought up individual accounts, rendered affectively, often through the real, physical, experience and display of emotion, when speaking about seemingly factual, statistical pieces of information about any of these issues.

Yet, the complexities around the way anonymity works is worth bearing in mind. Many mothers had spoken of the value of being pseudonymous or anonymous and being able to speak to just about anyone online about perinatal difficulties precisely because of never potentially having to meet them. But equally, they also spoke, sometimes even the same person who might value public forum pseudonymity, of the value of small-scale online groups – particularly WhatsApp groups – as very useful resources, propped up by offline meetups and more lasting connections. In these instances, they spoke of the value of being able to be oneself and open, which a pseudonymous experience on a public forum might not facilitate. And yet, even within these groups, there seemed sometimes to be degrees of non-disclosure and self-censoring which were tied into broader discussions and discourses around morally weighted issues of the perinatal. These introduced nuances into the role of publicness and privateness, anonymity, pseudonymity and openness in disclosing emotional difficulties to do with the perinatal. Heeya, who I had introduced previously in this chapter, demonstrated the juxtaposition and simultaneity of these subtleties well, as she speaks to me about her with perinatal self-disclosure:

> I guess like when online people ... You know, you don't know the people so you can probably be a bit more honest with them than you might be with other people. I'm quite an honest person anyway so I'm quite open with my friends as I am with online people. But I guess you just have that you know, that security of maybe not being judged so much by someone you know as well ... I just think sometimes people can be a bit, when they don't know people, they can be a bit nastier can't they?
>
> Heeya

As Heeya elucidates, being pseudonymous or anonymous online can make mothers feel safe in terms of disclosing perinatal difficulties, but it can also make people feel like anybody could say anything from behind that very pseudonymous barrier, leaving oneself vulnerable to attack. Under conditions of the perinatal ideal, when, as Chapter 2 argued, all aspects and dimensions of the perinatal have become very intensely moralised within intensive mothering discourses, decisions to disclose or not are rendered doubly difficult, over and above the fraughtness of self-disclosure in any case (c.f. Das & Hodkinson, 2019), owing to the moralised nature of disagreements and debates that might unfold in the specific contexts of the perinatal. This renders anonymity, pseudonymity and openness particularly complex for perinatal self-disclosure, as these all produce mixed outcomes, it appears.

Many mothers noted that, when really isolated, anonymity or pseudonymity are issues of far less importance than offline meetups and personal contact which comes through getting to know a 'real person', as some said. The scalability function of social media, as Chambers put it (2016), was made use of by many mothers to carve out non-anonymous connections within which disclosure was 'appropriate', and nobody might hide behind the protection offered by a keyboard and screen. Charlotte found herself entirely isolated and depressed, with a new baby and no support network. She had a PhD but found herself coping with illness and a sudden stop to work, whilst being isolated in a new area. She had set up and been invited to a series of small, close WhatsApp groups, which began initially from public forums around specific perinatal topics. The space where these smaller groups began, she noted, was of importance:

> I guess these are forums that are set up specifically for you know … it's people who are exactly in the same place/phase(?) as me, and so they're kind of … they've already signed up to wanting to talk a lot about like (laughs) babies and things and you know not all my friends have children.
>
> Charlotte

Charlotte drew to my attention, not just the fact that mediated disclosure was easier, to people she barely knew, but also that, specifically themed spaces, clearly and overtly demarcated for disclosure and sharing in peer settings (such as depression support groups or feeding groups) are different in terms of the ties they establish and the intimacies they facilitate and shape as opposed to existing strong ties, where, on the face of it, disclosure should be easier, but the figuring out of appropriate moments and boundaries of disclosure is a task in itself. A similar account is provided by Rani, who spent the vast part of pregnancy coping with severe Hyperemesis Gravidarum – something she felt her family struggled to fully comprehend as it is often misunderstood as 'just morning sickness' when it is significantly debilitating:

> The Facebook group's really, the Hyperemesis group is people of all around the world who've got Hyperemesis, I think only a group of about 600 people, and you just compare notes, so I could write in there and say today I'm feeling like this and other people will say okay I've had that and I met another woman actually from Bedford, through here, which I didn't even know. I find Facebook is a bit more personal, because you can see that person's photo and they can add you in, I don't know, I preferred it.
>
> Rani

What made a difference for Rani, and what mattered significantly to her then, was that the functions of pseudonymity in online settings afforded protection to those taking sides in issues readily moralised, and thus rendered vulnerable those disclosing – and more 'personal' connections, where a photo could be seen made that person more real and she felt more able to connect to someone she felt she 'knew'. Glenda displays a similar narrative, with a clear focus on only disclosing to those who are predisposed to be non-judgmental and like-minded and those she felt she knew or could get to know personally:

> The groups, I think, if you find the right one for you that you fit in, again, it's fine. If not, then you're ... You can feel quite insecure. It's very hard to gauge someone's feelings by what they're writing, the same as a text message. There's no emotion. So they could saying before jokily, oh, yes, well done, you know. Or it could be well done, you did it. You just don't know. And I think that's the danger. The group for large families – I found it on Facebook. And it's been great. It's been a great support. You have to have four or more to join.
>
> Glenda

Glenda had set out to build a large family and had six children when we spoke, with a seventh planned. This opened her up, she said, to a significant degree of criticism, snide remarks or judgemental jokes on the size of her family. She too found specific closed non-anonymous groups more useful to be able to disclose difficulties, and hence establish valuable ties.

Anisa was a second-generation migrant mother from an African background, and whilst she did not have family locally, she had a very supportive and strongly connected network of sisters and a mother she adored living a short train ride away, and she had a fulfilling career she was eager to return to when we spoke. She had not experienced significant perinatal difficulties and was happy and feeling positive, she said, throughout. But she noticed on her WhatsApp new mothers' group subtle but definitely present degrees of self-censoring from those women who felt their experiences did not quite fit real or perceived dominant narratives of the perinatal:

> For my antenatal group from the hospital, we made a little WhatsApp group, just ... So there were a few people just before me. Like two or three weeks before. Most of them had ... Actually I think before me most of them were natural births. But one ... But it was almost after ... But I think people who had a caesarean seemed to hold off their announcements a little bit ... I'm not sure. Or whether it's just anxiety over having to have the caesarean. You know, was there something wrong with the baby? And not to announce it straight away. Because the ones that gave natural births, you know ...
>
> Anisa

So, as Anisa makes evident, even using such scalable functions of platforms and doing the emotional labour involved with figuring out when disclosure might be safe, the conditions of the perinatal ideal render inter-group conversations difficult and sometimes stilted. It seemed even in small-scale online groups such as WhatsApp, as below, which had a history of offline connection that self-disclosure might be halted or contained owing to regulatory and prohibitive nature of moralising discourse around the perinatal.

In this section of my findings, I suggested thus that the very nature of the perinatal and the wider structural, personal, physical reasons behind mothers seeking out a range of many online weak ties in this period invites attention to these weak and often temporally contained ties. Although relatively speaking the majority of these are indeed of short duration, the emotional and affective strength both positive and negative that these hold albeit ephemerally, particularly for women experiencing emotional difficulties, is substantial.

Newly forged online ties and the shaping of pre-existing offline ties

Apart from the lasting emotional significance, both positive and difficult, of temporally contained, ephemeral perinatal ties, both fieldwork and discussions on online forums revealed that many mothers found pre-existing offline, strong social ties challenged, changed and often discussed online in ways that then fed back to offline changes in expectations and demands, however small these were. My first finding here is that the challenges to pre-existing offline ties during the perinatal period, themselves down to already mediated, wider structural issues in conditions of the intensive mothering, led to the increased seeking out of ephemeral, but nonetheless affectively impactful, weaker tie connections online, some of which moved offline. But equally, discussions about these structural issues, including the amount of instrumental and material social support they could access, reshaped for many mothers their expectations of and approaches to these offline strong tie relationships. Mothers often asked online:

> ... how much help does your DH [dear husband] provide in the morning when you are on maternity leave?

These women were often those struggling with partners doing minimal childcare. Online discussions demonstrated advice and support weaving in broader discussions around gender, childcare and women's participation in the workforce, among other issues, which many mothers then fed back into discussions of domestic labour in their relationships, albeit with mixed outcomes. The same applied to women's expectations of healthcare professionals, and the demands they felt able to make on their time and attention and the advice given by them. Discussions of health visitor advice on infant feeding came up frequently on the Mumsnet infant feeding sub-board, which then often led women to seek out alternative sources of support – such as that provided by a long-term NCT infant feeding counsellor online in an informal capacity – but also, often, to go back to the offline care settings and to make stronger and better-argued demands. The percolation of information, support, advice and dialogue, outside of the boundaries of otherwise ephemeral online ties, is critical in this regard. When one mother, struggling perinatally but worried about the outcomes of being honest with healthcare providers, asks for advice online, the ensuing online discussions then reshape her approach to the healthcare support system for mothers and direct her to offline, face-to-face care. An instance of this mediating influence is captured below:

> Be honest with your health visitor. She is trained to deal with parents who have the feelings you describe and can help you get the help and support you need. She will not take your baby away.

Charlotte, who I had mentioned previously, talked through her strong, pre-established friendships, where she often spoke regularly to friends, she established how it was hard for her to disclose her struggles in these strong ties, because she sensed a social expectation to be positive and to talk about lighter, not deeper, matters. She articulated this clearly:

> I guess it's the thing that you don't want to like bother people too much I mean I do talk to my friends. I haven't really talked to them so much about kind of ... more personal things, which is funny because you know they're closer friends (than online connections).

Then, through the public forums on Mumsnet, she stumbled upon a People Nearby Application called Mush – for mothers to meet other mothers in the local area. She found it in her to join, post a message and wait for a response:

> Yeah, well I was lucky that a group of mums had already set up a group and they said, and they saw my post and said do you want to join? So they've got a Whatsapp group which, which is ... and then since then they've set up a Facebook group for events. ... I've met them a few times, I think that's really helped I think and like you say, I can feel really isolating. So it's been really nice and there's nor ... there's always someone on the Whatsapp group and there's always someone who you know wants to meet up and ... and you find things through other things.

This demonstrates how an offline absence of support networks around her, but also the genuine difficulties in disclosing problems to otherwise strong and healthy offline strong ties (c.f. Das & Hodkinson, 2019), led her to reach out a range of online public groups initially. Here, what is notable is that the shared solidarities of pseudonymous spaces online and the 'safety' of posting on People Nearby Applications to meet fellow mothers online first led her to a gradual, graded movement from these wider, public settings to smaller, niche and private groups, which eventually moved offline and carved out for her an offline support network of her choice.

My second point is about shifts in the nature of pre-existing offline ties in the perinatal period and the potential role of ephemeral online ties, or indeed, mediated communication and information made use of as 'resources' to shape offline ties, in this context. Ellison et al. (2007, p. 1146) note, "bonding social capital is found between individuals in tightly-knit, emotionally close relationships, such as family and close friends". In the context of perinatality, there seems to be a nostalgic and idealised value added to large networks of women around women. As Drentea and Moren-Cross note (2005), the medicalisation of what was once "women's knowledge" takes mothering even further away from women's circles, leaving mothers more socially isolated. But, as fieldwork and online data demonstrated, particularly, although not solely, for migrant mothers, large support networks on the ground might, in many cases, perinatally, emerge to be constraining, crowding or not understanding enough in comparison to online communities (which of course, as I have shown above, are themselves far from homogenously empowering spaces).

Moumita, a first-generation migrant Bengali mother in the U.K., explains how her in-laws did not, owing to 'family and cultural norms', permit her to invite her own family to visit or stay with her, to provide crucial perinatal support. She was living in a village in India when she entered into an arranged marriage with a food factory worker living in a U.K. city, who was originally from India. She arrived in the U.K. with no family of her own and, unexpectedly for her, found herself pregnant within two months of her arrival. She had strong, warm relationships with people back in India, but was unable to invite any of them over owing to her husband's family in the U.K. refusing to let her do so. In theory, Moumita was surrounded by a network of relatives (her husband's family), but in practice, she was significantly isolated, her broken English in the way of her being able to access any meaningful amount of resources both on and offline:

> Yes, I go on the Pampers website and just read what happened. And after born, I read what happened, which month I need to give him food and everything. I don't know what is the water break and everything. I read and I tell my aunty and others in india. I WhatsApp or Skype as well.
>
> Moumita

Moumita spoke to me about how she used limited information she could find on nappy websites to piece together the basics of what labour might look like, or what terms such as *waters breaking* actually mean. She would then use things she had read online in her WhatsApp and Skype calls back to India, filling gaps in information, establishing her own expertise and agency in her own eyes, in these conversations as she transmitted information back to female relatives back home, whilst being surrounded by a large but unsupportive offline network of in-laws in a country very foreign to her.

A similar story, in some ways, is reported by Vanini. Like Moumita, she is of Indian heritage and living in the U.K., but unlike Moumita, she is surrounded by warm, supportive and helpful offline ties and a largely functioning on-ground network and thus had a low need for emotional support. What she missed and needed though was up-to-date information for her to feel in control and empowered through her own perinatal journey riddled with hyperemesis which needed hospitalisation and a birth which went very badly wrong. She needed information on all of this to circulate through her own offline networks from where she suspected a range of pressures and wrong information were making their way to her. Whilst what she needed on the surface was information, but as an extension of my earlier point in this chapter, the information was not simply information alone. It was needed, also, to mediate her existing strong, offline ties, to establish her authority and expertise and help her on-the-ground networks work better for her. And hence, information seeking through apps was regularly used by her to fill gaps in on ground networks to help them work even better perinatally.

Shamima, who arrived in the U.K. to stay with her new husband and immediately found herself having two children, both born with significant special needs and born through complex and traumatic labours, found it difficult to speak to me in a house full of relatives offering her support with material aspects of the day-to-day, but from whom she says she had to hide her perinatal emotional difficulties. She relied on her husband's income to buy phone scratch cards to call distant relatives instead, while she managed a household and looked after a tube-fed baby at home:

> I used to buy cards to call Bangladesh. You have phone Lycamobile Lebara, these phone and these. And before that when these I used to use cards to call Bangladesh. If you buy one card one pound you get 200 minutes or something.
>
> Shamima

While for native British mothers, and equally for migrant mothers from professional and affluent backgrounds, the benefits and risks of digitally mediated social ties emerged to be comparable, migrant mothers from less affluent socio-economic groups showed few online ties owing to not accessing these spaces, although they reported feelings of isolation and being alone while in a crowd and even feeling watched by large extended families. This is echoed by findings on Polish migrants from Ryan (2011), who notes that the greatest gendered networking seemed to emerge around childcare, and despite migrant mothers engaging in childcare-centred ethnic, local networks, these did not necessarily amount to sustaining, emotionally supportive, strongly bonded rapports.

Nasreen, originally from Bangladesh had three children aged 11, 6 and 2, when we spoke and described herself as a busy housewife at the moment. She had done a degree in commerce and her partner was an academic. She came from what she called a traditional Muslim family. Growing up, she said, speaking about birth was considered embarrassing and taboo, but she still managed to figure out that her mother's experiences were always a struggle with all her pregnancies. When Nasreen got pregnant with her third child, she wanted to figure out a way to be more in control of how birth and perinatality went for her, from labour to breastfeeding, and she started looking up resources online. Whilst she established very quickly from a range of videos and online groups that she wanted to have a natural birth and that she wanted to exclusively breastfeed, she encountered, within her relationship, some resistance to some of her ideas – for instance, to have a natural birth at home:

> Yes, I looked up the hypnotherapy online what that was all about ... And that helped me ... it reassured me to think it is possible. I think having hope makes such a difference. My husband thought it was really ... He kept rolling his eyes every time he walked in and heard me listen to the videos. He'd be, oh, my God, and walked out the room again. But he had to listen to it in the car on the way there. And he had to listen to it in there. Otherwise, throughout it, it was me really taking charge. Yes, it was me taking charge. I wanted to take charge of my own body, and my own way of having my experience. I wanted to be the main person in charge of it.

The use of these mediated materials to open up dialogue and negotiate positions in her relationship within the context of what she described as a 'traditionally' gendered family is significant here. The widespread belief within her family was that hospital was safest, and yet, Nasreen wanted to argue that, within what functioned quite well as largely warm and supportive offline ties, she had found evidence that home births and natural births are perfectly safe too. She made use of a range of hypnobirthing video material to try to carve out a space in her relationship where she could make a case for natural births, so to speak, within wider resistance. As it turned out, they decided to 'avoid the mess' of a birth at home, but she carried a range of objects from home, including the 'flower of Fatima' for good luck, and a range of tapes and YouTube videos to her birthing centre where she felt in control and had the birth she wanted.

Gaps in offline support and inadequacies in offline ties emerge for many reasons, as above, sometimes owing to gendered norms of childcare, sometimes to cultural taboos around mental health, sometimes to pressures on NHS-provided support settings or sometimes, as a professional, qualified mother feeling very depressed on maternity leave explains, owing to high levels of isolation from like-minded others. People nearby applications such as 'Mush' are increasingly made use of, as I discovered through fieldwork, to counter this last. These aspects of online ties all involved the material aspects of the perinatal, related to wide structural issues around gendered childcare roles, the physical difficulties of the perinatal and often contrasting intergenerational perspectives and attitudes to perinatal mental health issues. My central argument in this section has thus been that the material and emotional roles of traditionally held-to-be-important offline maternal support networks of mothers are renegotiated, repositioned and even by-passed through online ties, feeding, in general, into long-standing findings around the mutual shaping of the online and offline.

Discussion

In this chapter, I have sought to investigate the roles played by the perinatal ideal within digitally mediated interpersonal connections in the perinatal period. I have argued that these ties have complex positive and less than positive nuances, generating inclusions and exclusions which link to the moralised nature of conversations around mothering and good mothering in the perinatal. I have unpacked this core argument in a set of steps, positing first that online information seeking, in both one-way and interpersonal contexts, is complex in terms of perinatal well-being, because information itself is morally weighted and as such, information sits embedded within a normative and regulatory discourse. Because the perinatal – like much of rest of parenthood – is morally weighted in conditions of the perinatal ideal, which feed out of the imperative on women to mother intensively, no information, which in itself is graded and nuanced in its forms and garbs, is ever purely information and becomes affectively loaded. Information itself comes in many forms and shapes, and lines are blurred between formal and informal information and whether it appears in interactive settings or encountered as stand-alone information, it is never quite just information. I have gone on to discuss how multiple ephemeral ties are digitally mediated and set up during the perinatal period, a time frame which links to an 'acute/temporary' stage in parenthood, corresponding perhaps to similar time-contained acute, intense periods in other situations. These mediated ties might well in the long run be temporally inexpensive, but they are often affectively expensive in the here and the now, and equally, potentially tied into long-term memories owing to the precise social-cultural politics of intensive motherhood and the moral weighting of discourses and information. This affective strength despite temporal ephemerality is achieved, amongst other things, through self-disclosure, I suggested, which occupies a strange public-private interface on many online spaces, for instance, on Twitter.

I have also noted that maternal self-disclosure in online even anonymous communities might often be restricted and guarded owing to normative expectations placed on what is acceptable to disclose. But overall, I have argued that temporally transient, digitally mediated ties may have profound in-the-moment as well as long-standing emotional significance owing to the very nature of the perinatal. I suggested then that these ties weave themselves into offline structures, often leading to alterations in how people function in offline relationships, but also often bypasses offline rapports which may seemingly seem supportive but, in fact, may well not be so.

These findings also drew attention to the juxtaposition of the positive/emancipatory and negative/restraining aspects of digitally mediated maternal relationships rather than a dramatic disclosure of an either/or picture, drawing out the complex role of these online interpersonal connections in maternal well-being. I brought together sociological research on mediated interpersonal relationships as well as theorisations of the maternal in the context of perinatality, to carry both these conceptual avenues into consideration of the mutually shaping and embedded nature of media, technologies and the social world. The aim was not to promise dramatic or necessarily straightforward tools with which to make sense of mediated interpersonal relationships developed during the perinatal, but to suggest instead that the findings presented take forward the conversation, both on digital sites and maternity, and on perinatal well-being that has largely, until now, been studied in its offline contexts.

Note

1 A version of this chapter has previously been published as Das, R. (2018d). Temporally inexpensive, affectively expensive: Digitally-mediated maternal interpersonal ties in the perinatal months. *Communication Culture & Critique, 11*(4), 586–603.

6 Perinatal anxiety and its mediated social shaping

Up till now, this book has focused on interpersonal ties, talk and discussions and amateur video work as sites through which to look at the perinatal ideal as a mediated, intense and moralising ideology in contemporary digital societies, deriving out of the logics of intensive motherhood. In this chapter, I carry forward these issues to consider perinatal anxiety – perhaps the most 'visible' perinatal issue (within the broader framework of postnatal depression) that mothers are screened for and that appears with some regularity in media discourse. Maternal anxiety, particularly in the perinatal period before and after childbirth, has long interested professionals, the popular press and the public, usually as an individualised, clinical condition, which is linked via discourses of real and inferred blame to its impacts on the fetus/infant. Drawing upon interviews with mothers, I problematise this and argue that in contemporary digital societies, we must study perinatal anxiety in a mediated, sociological framework, complementing the locus of attention from mothers treated as individuals alone, to broader societal structures and conditions, all of which are mediated. I present my findings in two strands. First, I speak of the red herring of infant well-being, where I demonstrate how, in digital societies, perinatal anxiety often manifests, finds reassurance and is produced and maintained in the guise of highly specific infant well-being related issues, but is essentially rooted in ideals and ideologies surrounding mother blame. Second, I focus on the nuances and complexities of peer-to-peer support, where I scrutinise resources intended to support in the much spoken-about world of online peer-to-peer networks, which do indeed ease and provide support but in more subtle ways, often also maintain the conditions for anxiety by responsibilising mothers. I suggest we step away from individualised, pathologised, blame discourses of anxiety by focusing attention on the infrastructures of anxiety in contemporary mediated societies.

Perinatal anxiety often finds itself at the centre of popular and policy interest, ordinarily through a focus on 'maternal depression' (NCT, 2017). This chapter does not suggest that all maternal anxiety is solely sociologically shaped or indeed that clinical dimensions of anxiety are somehow in opposition to or less important than its social shaping. Indeed, it is arguably very important, in many instances, to find a diagnosis which offers clinical support, partly for the support itself, but also for the sense of liberation, emancipation and agency that might come through a formal diagnosis. This chapter does not disagree with any of this. Rather, the argument is that we approach perinatal anxiety through a lens which is broader than the individual and the solely clinical, locating it within contemporary structural logics of the maternal. Doubtless, also, not all mothers or mothers-to-be are anxious, and not all of those who are turn to the world of the online and indeed those that fall into both these categories are not to the same degree guided by discourses of mother blame. This chapter focuses specifically on the messy, mediated experiences of maternal anxiety of those who did experience various degrees of this, in my project, and it attempts to tease out the wider structures within which their experiences sit. I draw upon interviews with new mothers in the U.K., and on occasion, a weekly Twitter discussion hour on postnatal depression to explore the digitally mediated, sociological workings of maternal anxiety. The nitty-gritty of the perinatal everyday – from midnight searches online for breastfeeding positions, encountering nuanced discourses and often exclusive cliques of online peer-to-peer support, to seeking validation online (and struggling to find it) when switching feeding methods, for instance – all weave seamlessly across the offline and the online, blending the two, increasingly unnoticeably. It is important that we step away from historically entrenched swings between euphoric hope and moralising panic around digital technologies, particularly in the context of health (c.f. Lupton, 2016), but rather make sense of the ways in which maternal online communication, itself shaped by and shaping the structural conditions within which it operates, sometimes alleviates, sometimes worsens, increasingly shapes and always mediates the ways in which anxiety functions in contemporary mediated societies. The two cross-cutting arguments here are that, first, the perinatal ideal shapes maternal anxiety as opposed to solely pathologising/individualising discourses, and second, the mediated communication is an integral part of such a process, helping, hindering, but always shaping these structural conditions.

The cultural coding of maternal anxiety

Maternal anxiety comes with a heavy set of cultural codes attached to it in both lay and expert discourse. As previous chapters have noted, there has recently been a proliferation of mothers using social media, for instances, blogs, microblogs or social networking sites (c.f. Lopez, 2009), to express themselves, enabling mutual support and feedback on individual experiences of anxiety (Das, 2017, 2018). Some of this resorts to self-blame and guilt – as a blogger says, anxiety makes you an angry mom. Popular media seem to culturally code anxiety in such a way that it and the mothers associated with it are presented as a threat to infant well-being, with implications of mother blame. One source says babies of anxious mothers focus on threats (Bohn, 2017), a broadsheet declares that anxious mothers may disrupt infants' sleep (Smith, 2012), a tabloid says anxiety is 'catching' and may pass on to children (Hope, 2015), a leading news agency headlines that babies of anxious mothers are more likely to cry excessively (Lehman, 2014).

This set of codes corresponds with extensive expert discourse which measures the impact of maternal perinatal anxiety on infants, manufacturing individual women as units through which to understand anxiety and prioritising infants over rather than alongside mothers in the process. Highly cited chapters in psychology and wider biomedical literature typically links maternal anxiety to children's emotional/behavioural problems beyond infancy (O'Connor et al., 2002), fetal development (Van den Bergh et al., 2005), anxiety in older children (Van den Bergh & Marcoen, 2004), infant social engagement (Feldman et al., 2009), amongst others.

Across both sets of discourses, expert and lay, then we see maternal anxiety bringing with it the heavy baggage of its impact on the fetus, infant and child. At the heart of this cultural coding lies, first, the eternal inseparability of mother and child, unproblematically uniting woman and the unborn, the infant and the child, and second, imaginations of the child as society's hopes for its future. This is succinctly grasped by Parker (1997) who considers how the notion of change and development, which occurs rapidly in perinatality, for the foetus/infant, is grasped by ever newer and intricate technologies (c.f. Fage-Butler, 2017) and is always conceptualised in terms of the infant rather than the mother. Maternal anxiety thus becomes a 'burden' in popular discourse for the future adult, the future older child, the infant of today – on whom society's hopes are pinned – and thus fits neatly into being regarded as a problem for everyone in society but understood and needing resolution at the level of the individual mother. At this level, it begins to appear in awareness raising and public policy spaces as individual mothers needing help and support (NCT, 2017), which they doubtless do, and where austerity regimes are delivering lethal blows to the U.K. National Health Services' capacity to deliver appropriate support and care (DoH, 2011).

So, we might conclude then that there are perhaps four facets of maternal anxiety, similar to Lupton's account of the technico-scientific perspective on risk (1998) where such anxiety is objective, measurable and causal. First, the discourse recounted above naturalises perinatal anxiety as pathologised and something to be studied as a clinical condition alone (which it might very often be, but perhaps rarely ever alone so). Second, it is individualised – the individual woman is always the unit of making sense of it at most levels of analysis and support. Third, it is embedded in blame discourse – clinical literature studies its impacts on fetus and infant, and popular literature frequently established causal links between mother's anxiety and fetal/infant behaviour. And fourth, it is always understood in fetal/infant terms – measured in timelines relating to the child, supported/checked in timelines appropriate to the child and support offered in group settings involving the child (baby massage groups in the U.K., for instance).

Relevant to this focus on maternal perinatal emotional well-being, sociological scholarship has frequently looked at anxious parents and parental anxiety as part of discussions of risk and risk management in risk societies (c.f. Furedi, 2006b; Pain, 2006). This literature has critiqued how, in contemporary societies, the role of a parent has become the role of a risk manager, and much like an 'ideal' citizen, the 'ideal' parent is ever vigilant and always engaged in risk anticipation, management and harm avoidance. Here, parental anxiety, like other anxieties, might be considered to be a response to a world fraught with risks around myriad things from infant feeding (Faircloth, 2013) to food consumption (Keenan & Stapleton, 2010; Klinnert & Robinson, 2008). These discourses speak essentially to the arrival of the logic of 'perfection' where both parent and child must be perfect – perfectly vigilant parents parenting perfect children (Henderson et al., 2016; Williams et al., 2013). The risk society (Beck, 1992; Giddens, 1991b) and risk management inroad into anxiety has been further nuanced with socio-cultural approaches to risk as situated (c.f. Henwood et al., 2008), and socio-culturally contextualised and shaped (c.f. Tulloch & Lupton, 2003), considering the messy and fluid relationships between emotion and risk (c.f. Lupton on the emotion-risk assemblage, 2012a) and how both are fluid, in flux and embodied. Yet, we know little about the ways in which maternal anxiety or more specifically perinatal anxiety functions as an emotion. We know little about the material spaces it traverses, the project of the self it is messily located within and the societal structures and relations which produce and maintain it as a heavily culturally coded concept.

This means approaching the myriad struggles and pressures of perinatality this book speaks of, including healthcare systems and public understanding of perinatal difficulties and anxieties as problems that begin and end at the level of the individual mother, in a framework which moves beyond an individualised and largely blame based causal approach to perinatal and maternal difficulties, because this contributes to and arises out of the inseparability of mother and child that underlies the logic of intensive motherhood (Hays, 1998). As Theodorou and Spyrou (2013) note:

> anxiety, in this sense, is fundamental to the modern-day maternal project: to be a proper and good mother is to be anxious; to be without anxiety is to lack the motivation to address the risks inherent in having a baby. (p. 82)

The red herring of infant well-being

I suggest in this strand of my findings that perinatal anxiety manifests as acute anxieties on specific matters to do with infant health and well-being. Myriad apps and devices are designed to apparently alleviate but actually maintain such queries. A variety of support forums provide reassurance and once again, relief at the level of queries on infant well-being. But these distract and divert attention from the core issue: the damages to maternal sense of self within the logics of the perinatal ideal. My fundamental argument in what follows is that, in the vast majority of conversations on anxiety, it seemed that the highly meticulous fundamentals of fetal and infant well-being discussed at length worked perhaps as camouflages, carrying our discussions into accounts of practical worries, regrets, preparations and seeking reassurance. And yet, these all emerged to be embedded within a snare of intersecting, mediated structures and ties which manufactured the material and symbolic circumstances for the anxiety in the first place.

Violetta, who had a difficult pregnancy and birth, spoke to me at length about her online research done about miscarriages and neonatal loss. She herself works in healthcare for the NHS and supports people with drug and alcohol addiction. She had clear ideas about the need to establish a marriage first before having children and more particularly, she was intent on not having children too late (in her mind, having a first child at 30, which was her own position, was too late). Without being specific about any particular media text or online discussion, she emphasised the role of perfect narratives on "what you see around you on television really" which was:

> just that you got married in your early 20's; you had children when you were 25 and this house just magically appeared from somewhere and that you had money and a fulltime job. So all very, kind of, unrealistic, really.

Despite the recognition and critique of these representations as 'unrealistic', this is what she herself aspired to, drawing attention to the range of (mediated) and largely heteronormative structures her own dreams were operating within and against. But, importantly for her, her mother losing a child owing to what her mother put down as an aging maternal body played repeatedly on her mind. She noted that her mother "very much felt to herself that she'd left it too long between having children and that's why her body rejected the baby". When Violetta talked through her own antenatal anxieties with me, the possibilities of her womb rejecting the baby and violating the aspirations she was both critical of and adhering to were high, and the research she did fed back to her mother's stories and worries around neonatal loss:

> I did loads of online research on like mothers' age at getting pregnant and baby health. And it was all true – I was going to be too old. My mum had always put the fact she'd lost the baby down to the fact that there was 15 years between me and my brother. I was really worried, you know, I was kind of getting too old.
>
> Violetta

In the previous chapter, I had described Violetta's interfaces with online hypnobirthing material and practitioners. When encountering the media material around hypnobirthing, she found herself ashamed, embarrassed and feeling like a failure about her first birth, as the material outlined clearly to her that any birth that was not entirely 'natural' was wrong. She told me, in tears, about a video she watched as part of her course: "one of the videos she showed me through the hypnobirthing, one of the people actually described, you know, not wanting to have given birth to a drugged-up baby and I just wept because with (baby's name) I had pethidine". She went on to say:

> I did end up having forceps delivery and then ... I think if I would, kind of, been living in my own little world; I think I would have been able to have lived with it but hearing people going ... I don't want a drugged-up, dead baby or when people are like ... I didn't use any drugs when I had a baby and being super proud of it. And you start to think about yourself and thinking ... Oh, crikey. It makes you feel wrong.
>
> Violetta

Violetta's case, then, elucidates a range of points around perinatal anxiety, which, whilst expressing itself as being firmly focused on what is apparently best for the foetus and best for the baby, is tied intensely and inherently to a range of mediated structures which place great and ultimate responsibility on the mother and the mother's body, as chapters 3 and 4 outlined. Her experiences of anxiety seemed to feed out of a nexus of forces, some handed down through generational ties, some feeding into and out of broader gendered societal perceptions of women's bodies, age and fertility, but all in one way or another operating in mediated communicative conditions, with the curation and circulation of highly loaded and meaningful rhetoric and imagery.

Leticia gave birth and lost a baby to circumstances she could never find out about, an unresolved mystery forever, whilst in Kenya. Her experiences in Kenya were traumatic in myriad ways, and when she came to the U.K. and received antenatal care for her subsequent child, she recalled feeling both 'spoilt' and thoroughly daunted. Leticia has grown up in Kenya, where she says she did not know how tough things had been for her, "until I came to the UK. I just thought it was normal; it was the norm, that's how you live. You wake up, you do this; that's the life". When she lost her baby in Kenya, she found no support from either her own family or her in-laws. Even her mother, she says:

> never spoke to me about the dead baby, nothing. She would come and find me crying because we lived in the same compound. She would find me crying; she would never even care why I'm crying, even ask

> me or nothing. And the stuff that I had bought for baby, when she was coming to get me from hospital she took everything away from me. Yes, so it was horrible.

The sheer palpable difference between Kenya and the U.K. led to a thorough transformation as she described it and she found herself delving into the world of birth-training courses, online material and myriad apps to track and monitor her new fetus' development, but also to research how to do her best by her. One of the outcomes of this newfound world of both comfort and information was that she experienced perinatal anxiety twice over – first, managing herself and her actions minutely, for the intended welfare of her baby – for instance, modifying the sound levels of music she listened to while pregnant, and second, regretting over and again her perceived lack of preparedness about the baby she lost, wondering and worrying about if and how she had failed that baby by not preparing enough. She said, after coming to the U.K.:

> I was also reading books and, knowing that ... how to behave and how it's affecting my child. Knowing that stressing myself is affecting my child; knowing that even screaming or whatever ... And I knew that if I play loud music it's ... She's going to like it. She loves music because I used to play loud music to her. Yes, so it was really different but that was the ... That is the positive side of difference but there is a negative side, in the nascence that I'm more informed; I know neglect when I see it which, with my first one I didn't know. I didn't know neglect; I thought this is how things are run and I didn't question it ...
>
> Leyla

A version of pressure handed down across generations, similar to Violetta's story previously, is also visible in Leyla's account:

> She's got four, and she did, my mum had to give birth to a stillborn. She would have had five. But yes, every single one of them was natural. It was just gas and air, there was nothing else at all. It was failure to do it properly, as a woman should ... I didn't even do the labour properly.
>
> Leyla

Leyla spoke of both antenatal and postnatal anxiety around a variety of infant well-being related matters, but the topic we kept returning to is about 'giving birth the right way'. Her mother is far away and yet always present in her mind, and forms part of her referential framework – a web of affective codes she accesses, which tells her that she performed birth wrong, and potentially these trickle into myriad, specific postnatality related anxious feelings about getting other things wrong. She demonstrates throughout that her limited engagement with the digital is firmly embedded within these lived and handed-down experiences and emotions of the perinatal, spanning overlapping cultures, but also that these frame and position her own past and her actions in her own past whilst elsewhere as somehow inadequate and linked to her baby's death.

Charmaine spoke to me whilst doing a PhD and having had a baby recently, for the first time. She had planned a home birth, but complications during labour meant that the baby was born in hospital. She got involved with offline and online hypnobirthing material and training and said, "I was not afraid of it at all. I wasn't dreading it. I think because I was so convinced from having practiced so much ... I really wanted to make sure I did everything I could to achieve that natural birth". But as she recounted her actual labour experiences she spoke of surprise, then shock and then a feeling of failure, and a rising sense of anxiety as labour progressed, not because of any supposed fear of birth, but rather the growing sensation that the sensation she was feeling – pain – was an indicator in itself that she had done something wrong and the natural birth she needed to achieve was not quite going well:

> It was very uncomfortable. It was very sharp. It was very strong. So when I ... So that broke my concentration a lot. When ... If I ... If I was expecting pain, I think I would have dealt with it in a completely different way, but because I was convinced that I ... That it wasn't going to be quite like that, I started feeling that something was not right. I wasn't doing things right, which is stupid, obviously, because there is no right or wrong.
>
> Charmaine

Charmaine met a caring and kind natural birthing instructor, who led her into a set of discourses which idealise and valorise a seemingly pain-free birth as a woman's ambition and great achievement. This instance of anxiety is particularly valuable for it deals with the sense of anxiety during the very process of giving birth. In contrast to what one might expect, however, the anxiety here has less to do with any fear of birthing and more to do with standards for one's own birthing self. I draw attention to the subtle undertone of self-blame even when recounting and remembering the lived experiences of her labour in the quote below:

> There was a lot, a lot of, I think, you know, in my head, there was a lot of disappointment at that point, sort of disillusionment, that things weren't going as quite as I had planned. I think I was quite naïve in the sense that I'm sure hypnobirthing works for a lot of people, but for my personal mind-set or my personality, exactly what could have been a mismatch, but it didn't, it didn't, it didn't really work. I mean, I could relax, and I wasn't afraid, I mean, which I think is a bonus, and it might be, it might be that as I was practicing, I was not afraid. I was just really angry at myself and disappointed at myself that I wasn't doing it by the book.
>
> Charmaine

What we see in her narrative as she recounted the exact process of giving birth, sometimes welling up as she spoke to me, is not a fear of birth itself or a fear of the acute pain that giving birth involves. Even in the exact moments of going through the surges and waves of pain that labour involves, we see a real, palpable sense of wanting to 'do it right'. As she recounted her birth, it became evident that every step of a long and arduous multi-day birth was punctuated with ruminations about what she might have done wrong or what might have stood in the way of the perfect birth. The deeply physically sensate experience of anxiety here drew upon an encoding of the ideal birth she had gathered for herself through a year of practice and training in a specific natural birthing technique, ironically meant to have empowered her.

For Nritya, a second-generation migrant mother, whose parents and in-laws arrived from India and Kenya, an array of mediated sources, from leaflets and pamphlets, stories in the media and some information seeking online, led to a growing sense of anxiety around Caesarean sections. Her anxiety around the C-section led her to consider her birthing experience to not have been up to the mark. She framed her anxieties around a potential lack of bonding with her infant if a surgical birth was necessitated, but her words return once again to the maternal self, where the fear of not achieving a very particular experience, out of a process that is barely within one's control is evident:

> I just want it to be natural because I felt like having a baby by caesarean I was ... I was scared I wasn't going to bond. That was my biggest fear ... was the fact that I wanted the baby straight away on me ... Because I was like, you know, that's the whole experience. For me that was like the most natural way you could ever have a baby is ... That's the only way it'd be possible ... Because you kind of ... know, don't you, Obviously you being the mother you have that ... Don't you?
>
> Nritya

Taking the example of birth, as that is what many mothers spoke of, I remind readers once again that my critique is not placed at the level of whether or not a natural birth (however that is defined) is better for mothers and babies than one with interventions, particularly any manner of imposed and intrusive interventions, for decades of midwifery have now established beyond doubt that women's agency in birthing is of paramount importance. So, doubtless, my critique does not advocate, for instance, for a regression to obstetric control over and hyper-medicalisation of women's bodies. Rather, following the notion of the pendulum shift introduced in Chapter 4, I critique the heightened state of anxiety and self-responsibilisation that came across repeatedly from mothers in search of the ideal, for instance, the perfect, relaxed, pain-free birth – and by extension, the most natural forms as perceived for a variety of perinatal tasks and stages, from infant feeding to childcare decision. If this ideal is not reached, the ultimate return of guilt and blame on to the mother alone points us towards a return, I suggest, to gendered logics of mother blame feeding out of and maintaining a wider variety of (mediated) rhetoric and representations.

Instances of a practical, well-being oriented articulation of anxiety, leading back into roots of enormous maternal responsibilation in the perinatal years, comes across equally clearly in a weekly supportive platform for mothers with postnatal depression on Twitter:

> As someone with autism I find socialising difficult but I push past my anxiety as best I can so that my daughter doesn't 'learn' my autistic traits.
>
> Poster

Women self-disclose profoundly difficult experiences in the public platform of Twitter, generating a space on the hashtag that feels almost private. Here, we see myriad experiences of anxiety, including, as in the quote above, 'solutions' to this anxiety. Despite the undoubted supportiveness of the discourse, both the problems and the solutions seem to be driven by a strong sense of potential negative impact of maternal anxiety on infant well-being, as I had discussed previously in referring to popular culture rhetoric. Another mother demonstrates this clearly through presenting anxiety as something separate that acts in parallel to other things:

> Oh and when they were unwell, I am supposed to keep this human alive, omg I'm the responsible adult, no pressure! Coupled with anxiety it's hugely stressful.

This extends, perhaps, also to mothers and their own bodies in perinatality. Digital societies make possible newer avenues of comparison, tracking, monitoring, surveilling, managing and finding alleviation geared around the specificities of infant well-being. The most personal, private and intimate aspects of female bodies can be quantified through the daily monitoring of bodily temperatures, fluids, emotional states and then fed into a broader pool of data which will apparently improve insights and predictions of fertility and menstruation. As one mother said:

> I am fully in control of knowing when I am due on ... and then when I'm going to ovulate, so really convenient and keeping me in the loop about my own body ... but my temperature did not rise the way it was meant to, and this probably means another month and I have not conceived.

As scholars succinctly argue (Choe et al., 2014; Lupton, 2016; Mol, 2000 amongst others), these applications can encourage women to live in a permanent state of anxiety and close monitoring of their own bodies, perhaps even increasing anxiety rather than relieving it. I found in my conversations with women that they presented conflicting discourses around these invitations to self-monitor and self-regulate in the context of fertility and conception.

For Cathy, we spoke as she nursed her new baby. He was her second pregnancy, but her first baby because they had lost a baby the previous year at 12 weeks. Cathy recalled her pregnancy as being simultaneously full of worry and full of planning and fitness regimes. She elucidated how she was really worried that the birth wouldn't go the way she wanted it to. She said she liked to think she was quite healthy, and she used to play netball, run, did Pilates all the way through her pregnancy. She had a hardcore fitness plan that altered throughout her pregnancy. So, for instance, when she stopped netball when she was about 12 weeks because it was a contact sport, she replaced it with Aquafit. She was really keen to be really fit, because she said that she felt the fitter she was the more likely she was to get through it without needing help:

> It was very idealistic, a lot of people were quite, well, you do whatever you need to do. And whilst that was the case, and I was really, really, really nervous, and I didn't want caesarian. I would have probably done quite a lot to not have a caesarian. I think being fit and healthy, because that's what I thought in the first place, I think because I was fit, or tried to keep fit all the way through, I'd been really successful. I was really anxious that my fitness would not be good enough for the baby to be well at and after the birth you know?
>
> Cathy

So, Cathy's conversation with me revolved almost entirely around a selection of tracking approached to her physical fitness. We spoke of high impact exercise, regular runs, aerobics and a variety of sports, particularly in the run-up to giving birth. She organised for herself an entire array of sporting activities that she had carefully planned in order to prepare her body to be at its athletic best for labour. On probing, she revealed a deep-seated fear and, to an extent, disdain of the possibility of C-section. She expressed a view that whether or not a birth will become a C-section is entirely in the birthing woman's control, speaking to me of her sister-in-law who 'ended up with a C-section' and how she was surely unfit. Cathy's elaborate sporting routine was tied very evidently to her anxiety around achieving a natural birth for it was best for her baby, she said that she did not 'need help'. Once again, practicalities around infant well-being and changes to maternal responsibilities indicated a deeper-lying set of assumptions connected to the responsibilisation of mothers, which Cathy had put together from a wide variety of sources.

Online, on Twitter, there are anxious references often to the amount of milk collected or not in the collecting unit of a pump, or to the use of a monitor to monitor an infant's breath, following accounts of cot death or to nappies being filled enough or not. Offline, too, in countless conversations with mothers, where they were battling baby monitors, breast pumps, transitioning between breast and bottle or coping with the return to work from maternity leave, interviews would often veer into detailed conversations seemingly about objects, but essentially about discourses around good-enough and not good-enough mothering in reference to the intensiveness of the perinatal ideal.

In this section above, I distilled instances of maternal anxiety in antenatal, birthing and postnatal periods, nearly always presenting itself as logical, factual and clearly articulated concerns around infant and fetal well-being and doing the 'best thing'. All of motherhood, but the perinatal specifically through its focus on infant futures and infant well-being, permeates cultural policy, institutional discourse and lay talk, manufacturing the infant's enormous societal value as an integral part of future discourse (see also Alper, 2019) as inextricably tied to the mother, manufacturing the perinatal ideal. The interview experience in speaking about these anxieties would very often get into the detailed medical nitty-gritties of infant development and even maternal bodily health. And yet, more often than not, these very detailed nitty-gritties emerged to be smokescreens, acting like red herrings, taking the conversation into accounts of practical anxieties and reassurance seeking, when, on probing, it emerged that a wide web of overlapping, mediated institutions and relationships created the conditions for the anxiety in the first place.

Nuanced complexities of support systems and support rhetoric

In this strand of my findings I argue that perinatal anxiety – like myriad other conditions – increasingly finds useful spaces of online disclosure and support, amidst blame and shame discourses, as chapters 4 and 5 have shed light on. The growing culture of myriad online fora speak to institutional and societal pushes to 'find support', which places the burden on individual women and on peers who are themselves struggling, whilst offline sources of support through local, state-supported means, recede. And while blame discourses might be avoided if one is careful and vigilant online (itself a responsibility), peer and institutional support discourses double up as responsibilising discourse, often celebrating the 'great mother'.

Doubtless, like myriad other conditions and difficulties, burgeoning online support communities bring together many mothers who have access to these spaces (not something we must assume or take for granted, as Chapter 7 elucidates). An array of evidence has, by now, accumulated on the value, for those struggling with mental health difficulties, of peer-to-peer support in online communities (see Melling & Houget-Pincham, 2011, for a review).

Indeed, maternal anxiety achieves reassurance and positive outcomes in support communities, perhaps rendered particularly visible in the online spaces it occupies. Digital technologies enable fluidity of movement across myriad overlapping spaces, with myriad un/known bodies appearing simultaneously, propping up an affective network which both relieves and maintains perinatal anxiety. New, intangible objects and acts – products of mediation – a virtual 'pub' or supportive emojis, the virtual breastfeeding lounge exemplifies the new socialities within which perinatal anxiety finds space and relief:

> This happened to me. Little one was 1 and a bit and I went to a baby class as my therapist said I should get out. So off I went anxiety through the roof. I walked in and looked at all the mums so happy and wondered why me and went in the toilet and cried the rest of it.
>
> poster

This tweet is an interesting account of how, in the first instance, the physical space of a seemingly anxiety-alleviating, private, offline baby group became an impossible space for this mother to occupy, who had undertaken a step to manage her anxiety. Yet, disclosing this overpowering experience in the online, intimate 'space' of a hashtag, while Twitter itself making such a space public, feeds into an environment of reciprocal emotional self-disclosure (Barak & Gluck-Ofri, 2007), rendering this space to be one where she lets go.

The hashtag for a supportive weekly chat itself gets used for myriad instances of support, of supportive memes, messages, artefacts involving art and creative writing 'going viral' amongst mothers. There is genuine solidarity which emerges from a tweet that says "I am a survivor of severe PND, PTSD, anxiety. Mum of 2 and now a mental health first aid instructor on a mission to raise awareness" or another mother who says she "shared (her) PND & Anxiety recovery story on Facebook Live last night. Catch the replay here". Here, as Ahmed notes (2004), 'feelings-in-common' are key. This is reflected also in work from the cultural geography of difficult emotions acting as connective tissue (Davidson & Milligan, 2004), where we might begin to think of perinatal anxiety as wielding and forging affective ties and generating senses of accomplishment in helping others and ones' own self work through these, as can be seen in these discussions.

I do not simply make the case that anxiety acts as a tool through which new mothers bond with each other, but I consider how the mediated collectivities Christine refers to below and indeed all manners of perinatal well-being peer support online emerge, because the very emotion of anxiety as articulated in the private-public space of a group or hashtag 'accomplishes' something. Christine recounted to me a difficult childhood with her mother and how her going on to having a child was an extension of her past childcare responsibilities for siblings growing up. She said that having a child herself didn't make much of a difference, because she never got to go out, just as she had had to look after her brother and sister. She decided to have an abortion for her first pregnancy, but says she regretted it every day and she spiralled into depression after that. She said:

> I thought it had all gone away and I thought all the feelings and everything had gone away because I never really noticed it. But then once I had him, he was planned, and ... I couldn't even tell you what went through my head, I couldn't go near him, I couldn't pick him up when he was crying, I just didn't want him around. And that was for at least the first two and a half, three months. So I got to the point where I wouldn't even open the curtains, I wouldn't get out of bed, people were ringing, I wouldn't answer my phone, I completely secluded myself, didn't want to talk to anyone, didn't want to go out, even going to the shops was, which was five minutes from me then, was a mission, complete mission.
>
> Christine

Christine, in that state of complete inability to step outside the house, chanced upon an online mothers' support group. Later, she found PND groups. From feeling like she was the only one going through such agony and that no one understands anything, it was very useful for her to see she was not alone:

> It was on one of the PND groups ... there's quite a lot of women that have put their heart out there and said what it's like, and I thought do you know what, I'm going to do it, it might help me within myself. I didn't even tell my family about it for a long time. Because I, I felt ashamed, I felt embarrassed.
>
> Christine

Just as it might generate discord and disconnection, misunderstood often in popular culture as fights between individual women (Das, 2018), it might produce mediated collectivities and new objects and spaces – the handhold, the sweet cup of tea, the lounge, the pub – not virtual spaces as in a whole different platform but affective spaces created just through words ... where the 'mediated appearance of others' – increased "awareness of the everyday lives and activities of significant others through the background presence of ubiquitous media environments" (Madianou, 2016, p. 1).

But, not all experiences take this route, and broader complexities about the burden of peer-to-peer support, on peers themselves, are themes I now turn to in what follows. Edna, when we spoke, was in the position of having two children under the age of two and had just had her contract terminated during her pregnancy. In addition, she had prior experience of depression with her first child, which she put down to the fact that she was in an unhealthy relationship at the time. She struggles to locate her perinatal anxiety within the boundaries of the pregnancy alone as, she notes, "it's hard to say I guess the depression was maybe due to the different areas of my life it affected ...". She also notes that she was unable to seek help when she had faced difficulties in the past, because "that comes with maturity, especially with mental health, you have to know that you're going through it before you can even seek help for it ...". So, for her second time round, whilst she was more aware of the implications of depression, she had a close friend, a nurse, who strongly believed it was hormonal alone and that it would settle soon. But it did not. Alongside therapy, Edna then ventured online to find peer-to-peer groups where she might find support for her anxiety, and indeed, she found a few of these straightaway. It was a postnatal depression support group on Facebook and her first thought was that it did not seem friendly. She struggled to articulate what precisely it was that made her feel unwelcome and she made a valuable argument about the inherent difficulties with seeking support from a group of mothers, who themselves are all in need of support, and presumably, given national trends and conditions relating to on the group postnatal support, might themselves be struggling to find what they need. The burden of listening, she articulated, was substantial, and thus, when everyone pours in their struggles, support is hard to find. So, Edna spoke of the difficulties associated with online peer-to-peer support communities, despite vast bodies of evidence outlining the myriad ways in which these offer camaraderie and benefits:

> I'm very ... particular with where I seek my advice from, knowing the fact that I am very emotional. Most of the time they're just literally set up by other mums. Which is good, it's good to have mum groups, but at the same time it can be sometimes more damaging than good, because they're also in their state of depression themselves ... the women were clearly severely depressed and lacked a real sense of being able to communicate politely with each other, so people were very angry and that came across in people's messages.
>
> Edna

Edna spoke of a minor disagreement between herself (while anxious) and another anxious new mother on the subject of a Chinese takeaway, where a seemingly mundane and trivial matter erupted into her having to leave the community. But her reflections draw out a wider point here about the increasing turn to peer-to-peer support communities, whether on or offline, amidst a general receding of state support in the postnatal period (DoH, 2011). On the one hand, as Edna notes, these communities are bottom-up communities of mutual support, which are useful in all manner of ways. But on the other hand, the burden of support here falls on the shoulders of those themselves direly in the need of support and all of whom have usually struggled to find resources or face-to-face professional support offline.

Direct evidence as to whether perinatal mothers are turning to these spaces because of on-the-ground lack of support elsewhere or whether they would be likely to do so anyway, is yet to be established, but interesting recent findings from the U.S.A. (c.f. Andersen & Parker-Ward, 2019) reveal clearly that, in response to the arrival of the Trump administration in 2016 and resultant uncertainties over maternity and wider healthcare service provision, the volume of maternity-related social media postings on Twitter rapidly shot up. So, the burdens Edna highlights find expression as 'wars' over trivial matters between individual mothers, but the circumstances which bring about a degree of reliance on such communities mean that the collective and the individual are both burdened in the task of finding and providing support when in an anxious and depressed state.

Sofia is one of five children and was born in Algeria, where she had a traumatic and difficult childhood. She has two children of mixed ethnic heritage and has had a history of anxiety through her own parenting journey. She describes a childhood of confusion, uncertainty and learning rapidly that she needed to fend for herself: "I grew up quite a confused person. But I did what I can to help myself growing up". She was born with some serious physical difficulties which were not treated when she was growing up, and she had various rounds of complex surgery once she was older and could arrange these for herself. Eventually, she found her emotional struggles getting in the way of work and she was made to leave work. She describes a history of abusive relationships, having children early, not having a supportive family around and she says, "although I knew it wasn't normal, I played normal until I was strong enough to leave and that was after I had my second child". Like Edna, this time round, she looked for support amidst peers:

> For me it's about using the resource, so using the internet and sharing your story with the right people in order to get what you think might work. I know what will work, but do I know how to get it, without telling the wrong people?
>
> Sofia

Sofia thinks the onus is on her as an individual to find the 'right people' to speak to, as she has always done, fending for herself since childhood, as wider structures – individuals, communities and institutions – failed her. And the account she shares is similar, as she outlines the impacts such interpersonal difficulties in peer-to-peer support communities online might have for a mother who is already anxious. She treats the Internet as a resource, but despite her acute need for disclosing and unburdening her anxieties to peers, past experiences have taught her that she must vet very carefully before she shares herself and her vulnerabilities.

But setting aside such structural issues around the difficulties which burden anxiety-related peer support communities, the very discourse of support itself merits attention. This has also recently been drawn attention to as a paradoxical relationship between support groups and the nuanced and mixed textures of actual, received support, where stigmatised groups may not actually find support from such communities (Yeshua-Katz & Hard, 2019). Extending this to the idea that support for some might not mean support for all, the discourse, availability and inclusivity of support groups merit attention. Charlotte has a PhD and was on a year off work on maternity leave when we spoke. She used to work in London, and whilst her partner continued his career, she found herself at home with an infant, isolated and struggling emotionally. Things were worsened by the fact that she had a diagnosed neurological condition which affected her maternity leave in the second trimester. She found it hard going because she had to end up working at home very early and not being able to go into the office. This became isolating and not knowing people around where she lived; she felt that she didn't really have a support network. She was referred to an online programme for some therapy, because appointments for offline face-to-face therapy were difficult to find and attend, but she says that she was so tired, she did not end up using it that much. It was at that point that she joined a Mumsnet group for people who were due in the same month as her, which then became a private Facebook group for a few of the posters who decided they were ready to shed their anonymity and get to know each other, and this then led to offline meetups. This graduated, graded approach to privacy and the movement from pseudonymity to openness worked for her:

> it's a private group, so … I guess it's nice because other people shared personal things, you know, it's been, everyone's been quite open on it, so I think that encourages you, and because it's a private, closed group it's kind of, you still feel like you've got some security.

Despite these benefits, Charlotte reports different experiences within such a supportive group for those mothers that felt excluded. I argue elsewhere in this book that all inclusions might function simultaneously as exclusions (Phoenix, 2019), and what Charlotte describes falls within this:

> I think there's quite a few mums you know suffer from anxiety and … in different ways … yeah, like body, worries about their body, also health … health issues. I think a lot of mums do end up a bit alone don't they? … I mean it is very emotional, you know, talking about you know there's some mothers who formula feed, some who breastfeed, and … there was one, there was one lady who suddenly left the group, and they think it might have been because they were saying things about … formula, and she kind of took it a bit personally.
>
> Charlotte

What Charlotte describes might easily of course be written off as the story of one individual in one group somewhere in England or even as a story of mothers competing with each other as individuals, as these things often are presented to be in wider public discourse. But a wider structural problem exists, where the fraughtness and tension in many similar online support communities for anxious or depressed mothers are twice burdened. First, they operate within a web of existing discourses of intensive mothering, and second, they must self-sustain and support each other when everyone is feeling fraught and nearly nobody has access to the levels of offline support that they might truly need. Such circumstances render online support communities a difficult, uneven and uncertain space for individual mothers like Sofia, who have interpreted the fraughtness of online encounters as having to do with them not having somehow spotted the right kind of peers. Harman et al. (2019) note similar things about conversations on feeding children and how feeding has become a site with heavy social and political load attached, where the 'good' mothering of 'priceless' children is under constant evaluation from a wide range of individuals, communities and institutions.

Kavya, a British Indian woman married to a white British man, was worried about her newborn daughter growing up not having any ethnic roots within the Indian community. So, they moved closer to her family, where she found herself surprised and getting increasingly lonely and feeling misunderstood. She says she initially did not think that she had PND and dismissed her difficulties as tiredness, particularly because in her own family nobody had spoken about mental health issues and she was aware of wide cultural stigmas and taboos around these matters, and had concluded that this was something that happened to others. A very helpful Health Visit urged her towards seeking peer support, in the broader context of NHS services being stretched, and she hesitantly reached out to the world of the online. Particularly, she reached out to Asian mothering groups online, when similar Asian spaces offline felt overwhelming and surveilling (Das, 2018) in the depths of paralysing anxiety, experienced these online spaces as simultaneously empowering and anxiety-inducing:

> On Bedford Mums or Recommended Asians, one of them, people have posted about their kids having issues with feeding or whatever. I've not wanted to post because I know a lot of my family are in that group as well, or I've got friends in that group, so I've just directly messaged them.
>
> Kavya

On the one hand, these spaces enabled her to be 'elsewhere' whilst on her sofa, unable to turn a key in a locked door, but on the other, they bore vestiges of offline relationships and policing structures around mothering practices in relation to weaning and infant food, meaning that she was unable to fully express herself. For many mothers in this project, offline and online blurred significantly in terms of anxiety, and the same spaces bore enormous amounts of blurring in terms of whether they meant relief or exacerbation from struggle and pain. Kavya spoke of joining groups such as Mums of North West London, Recommended Asians or Mums of Bedford to find some comfort she says through reading other people's posts similar to her circumstances rather than her having a discussion about her own. However, on one of these groups, she met a range of Indian relatives, some close and some distant, who began advising her publicly on the groups, speaking to her "as if I'm the little niece who's had a baby, rather than a fellow mum". Specifically, when she discussed her anxieties around infant feeding and weaning, she encountered disagreement and overt pressures to do things differently which spiralled her into cycles of self-doubt. But more importantly, she struggled as she tried to articulate to me how the support she found positioned her as a 'great Indian mother' and what that connoted to her in her own contexts:

> I was in a group for Asian mums when I was at the peak of my anxiety and depression. Yes they were supportive. But, I am not sure I was good enough by their standards. You are expected to do lots of home cooking, you're expected to keep a nice tidy home. Like that's what a good Asian mum does.
>
> Kavya

Kavya demonstrated the subtle pressures of 'support' discourse succinctly as she struggled to explain to me why an online community, which provides her great support through paralysing anxiety and debilitating depression, is the same community which 'boosts' her with a rhetoric of being a good Indian mother and a good Indian wife, which she knows places her under an inordinate degree of burden, maintaining the very anxiety she seeks alleviation for. Like Kavya, mothers often informed me that they found a valuable sense of fellowship online, which often spilled into offline friendships. Here, as findings in the following section will also indicate, valuable affective ties and bonds might emerge around the shared sense of anxiety and the sense of urgency and immediacy related to infant well-being related worries at all times of the night (Das, 2017, 2018). And yet, discourses of support that arise in many such communities offer reassurance, feedback and well-intentioned boosts which resort frequently to the trope of the good mother. Reassurances, when garbed thus, mobilise a degree of responsibilisation then by framing the yardstick and the goalposts as being a good mother – itself tied messily into complex and gendered discourses of the perinatal.

Marie, a Zimbabwean mother living in the U.K., also demonstrates, albeit in a different sense, cross-cutting structural pressures lie embedded within support and supportive structures, rendering support non-monolithic, nuanced and complex. Whilst Skype became a lifeline for Marie, with family back in Africa, it was through Skype that a series of misunderstandings and pressures were transmitted as to why Marie was not coping well on her own here in the U.K. with two high risk pregnancies. Marie was a first generation migrant mother, both of whose pregnancies had been classed as high risk, meaning that she had to be in hospital every two weeks with both pregnancies. She used a range of online resources for her second pregnancy, anxious not to repeat her son's suffering with colic. She was plagued by cross-cutting pressures between Africa and the U.K. Back in Zimbabwe, she felt nobody quite understood how hard it was to cope alone with high risk situations, "because they are all like a team, they work together. You know, there's somebody there to support you. So you don't really see how difficult it can be if you're on your own". But also, she encountered borders and immigration restrictions so much so that her "GP had offered to write a letter to the Home Office for me to be able to bring somebody over to help".

Online bonds seem to become particularly reinforced when they move offline – something evidenced also in women's accounts of using breastfeeding support groups which have a simultaneous online and offline presence. In many instances, women spoke of pressures and even intrusions from well-meaning offline support systems where they felt unable to explain themselves, which led them to look for support that was accessible and available online, which in turn, moved towards newer offline connections of support. But such support, as discussed previously, continues to be nuanced, embedded within and producing broader politics and logics of the perinatal ideal. Monica demonstrates complex sets of supportive discourses which leaves her bound to structural pressures in dual ways, cutting across the online and offline. Monica struggled to establish breastfeeding initially and found herself progressively anxious over her role as a mother, as she found herself at the receiving end of family pressure to switch to formula. Desperate for support, she found an online breastfeeding support group which very quickly resulted in offline meetups. But as she began to plan her return to work and wanted to stop breastfeeding by tapering it down, this group became progressively difficult for her, as it ramped up the support on her as a 'great mum' to continue to feed to the WHO recommend two years, leaving her confused as to why the texture of support no longer felt fully supportive. As Monica, a mother who initially struggled to establish breastfeeding, said to me:

> My mother and mother-in-law both were insisting that my daughter was not gaining weight fast. I started exploring the Facebook groups on breastfeeding support and went along to one of their summer picnics that I realized that actually she is okay ... But then when it was time I wanted to stop feeding, ... I'm not sure ... yes supportive, maybe but ...
>
> Monica

What happens then is interesting, as the very discourses of support online, which moved offline and which provided relief and alleviation from existing cultures of offline familial pressures, ends up subtly responsibilising and producing newer conditions of anxiety and mother blame, drawing our attention once again to the crux and nature of discourses of support as themselves simultaneously holding the possibilities to become discourses of responsibilisation through which the perinatal ideal continues to be articulated. Thus, we might consider the ways in which mediated networks of physical, material objects and spaces become affectively meaningful for maternal anxiety. The seemingly endless wait at a Health Visitors' clinic for a baby weigh in of a baby struggling to gain weight, or the object of a forceps arriving at the end of a planned 'natural' birth which became an instrumentally assisted one or the whirring of a breast pump which does not seem to be extracting much milk might become loaded and encoded with affective power, and both begin to speak to a notion of a mother not being 'enough' or not being 'good-enough'. Mothers do not seem to experience support as a stable, homogenous, uniform category, as it often makes visible uncomfortable realities of the wider political, economic, societal, cultural contexts within which early motherhood sits. It spills fluidly across online and offline spaces as mothers encounter, and are both supported and triggered by a range of actors, objects and institutions in the process. So, the paradox here in digital societies is that they seem to alleviate perinatal anxiety by making support seem freely, anonymously, 24/7 available – and it often has myriad utilities. And, yet that support itself might over-responsibilise twice over. It creates a burden of self-support and peer support on individuals and communities struggling with perinatal anxiety as state support recedes. And even within the discourses of support, notwithstanding cliques of inclusivity and exclusivity, the rhetoric of support might often be built upon the 'great mother' paradigm, which subtly and often even unintentionally serves to burden and responsibilise.

Discussion

Standing on the shoulders of groundbreaking scholarship on parenting and risk (c.f. Furedi, 2006b; McVarish et al., 2013), it would be logical to conclude that maternal anxiety is socially shaped – and rooted in long-standing gendered discourses of intensive mothering (Hays, 1998), mother blame, the notion of fetal celebrity (Parker, 1997) and the associated notions of matricide, for clearly there are broad structural processes which underlie it. But these social structures and the actions of social actors, today, operate in a mediated world. This means that the fundamental texture of these structures is mediated in ways which shape them both materially and symbolically. The mediated shaping of these structures, norms, ideals cannot be comprehended by asking "does technology make mothers more or less anxious", for that is a futile question. The real question then is, *how do the arrival and uptake of newer technologies shape social conditions of anxiety, both materially and affectively?* Perinatal anxiety, although largely studied clinically and through the four cultural codes discussed in this chapter, was always sociological, but how, if at all, does digital mediation of the social world produce infrastructures through which perinatal anxiety is alleviated and exacerbated, produced, maintained and understood?

The discussions of structures shaping anxiety, which I have forwarded in this chapter, draw our attention to the notion of materiality (for instance, the physical architecture of a building), second, the affective, symbolic and discursive realms (for instance, the warm, fluid, unfixed events, conversations, actions that transpire in the building) and indeed the institutional, both formally and informally. Whilst it is indeed key to investigate the widespread materialities of these platforms of the perinatal as assemblages which profoundly alter the conditions of the perinatal, my far more rudimentary suggestion here is that a separation of the societal and the digital is untenable if we are to think about the social shaping of perinatal anxiety. This is because the infrastructure itself would be different – we would still have social actors in a social world, but the selective presentation of selves generating a timeline of who we appear to be, the curation of mothering images which symbolise perfection, the curation of entire timelines heavy with ideology, the visual cultures of representations of motherhood and maternal gaze, the 24/7 anonymity and immediacy of the simultaneous appearance of myriad others, the powerful and short-lived social ties that move fluidly across online and offline in their impact, even if people never meet, the new intimacies carved on a meetup app, the encountering of myriad other bodies and the pleasures and pains of these bodies across social networks – and we can no longer make sense of these ties, relationships, norms, discourses outside of frameworks of mediation. Likewise, how shall we understand the relationships between surveillance, monitoring, vigilance and perinatal anxiety without considering how the harnessing of anxiety by large-scale data harvesting corporations, manufacturing ever newer devices and apps? How do we unpack the societal maintenance of anxiety without considering the embedding of apps playing on the morally heavy eternal mother-child bond by companies promising the monitoring of fetal heartbeats, the curation of 3D scans on social media timelines generating imperatives to measure, surveil and most importantly, maintain the conditions of anxiety? So, materially, symbolically, affectively – those very social infrastructures shaping and maintaining perinatal anxiety – then would be different outside of frameworks of mediation.

At a time when significant gaps in care are emerging for perinatal mothers (DoH, 2011), at a time when great hopes and expectations are placed on digital health (c.f. Lupton, 2018; Rogers, 2015) and at a time when lay and expert discourse continues to position maternal anxiety as an individual condition within a body of conditions within postnatal depression and anxiety, this chapter suggests that we might turn fruitfully to the mediated everyday in order to make sense of maternal anxiety. In this sense, the perinatal ideal is an outcome and component of intensive motherhood which is rendered overwhelmingly visible in the perinatal years with its overt focus on fetal and infant well-being, measurements, scans and outcomes. I suggested here that the perinatal period, both owing to the physiological rapidity of infant development in a short time and owing to the deeply moralising discourses surrounding this, is a ripe ground for the notion of the perinatal ideal to permeate physical objects and spaces, manufacturing through the inseparability of mother and infant, a set of conditions which both produces and maintains maternal anxiety. Thus, it is only through an analysis of mediated, moralised structures of perinatality, including the social relations, interpersonal expressions, individual and group behaviour and the consequences arising out of this, we might begin to make sense of how maternal anxiety presents itself, how it functions and what it achieves.

Under frameworks of mediation, then we might consider the mutual shaping of the digital and anxiety at the level of individuals, communities and institutions, not making a case that the digital is distinct, for it is quite the opposite or that is provides magic solutions or conjures brand new conundrums. In discussing the mediation of perinatal anxiety in digital societies, I hope to have demonstrated that a range of complexities are emerging at individual, communal and institutional levels. At the level of the individual, it seems clear that the onus of seeking and finding (the right kind) of online support is increasingly on the anxious mother herself, as peer support seems but rarely is the utopian solution to receding state support. Also at the level of the individual, dataveillance through the latest devices and monitoring apps ensures that perinatal anxiety is the raw material needed to lubricate mechanisms of surveillance. Digital societies make possible newer avenues of comparison, tracking, monitoring, surveilling, managing and find alleviation geared around the specificities of infant well-being, but these are born out of and maintain perinatal anxiety within logics of intensive motherhood. At the communal level, support forums – in addition to exacerbating anxiety through blame discourses – often display subtle responsibilising messages through seemingly supportive discourse. Responses provided to anxious well-being related queries often present as loops focused on well-being which alleviate sometimes, but leaves larger question around mother blame and responsibilisation largely unaddressed. At the institutional level, a faith in peer support in digital societies might enable institutions to pass on responsibilities to struggling peers leaving key gaps unfilled offline.

I hope to have demonstrated in this chapter that the question can never be whether technology resolves or exacerbates perinatal anxiety, perhaps to the disappointment of those expecting dramatic answers in the realm of digital health. I hope to have shown that we need to focus on anxiety in a non-individualised, non-pathologised and non-mother blame framework – which is simultaneously sociological and mediated. So, sociologically, it seems imperative that we continue to unpack the structural conditions of mothering intensively in risk societies, which enable perinatal anxiety to be manufactured and maintained as individual women's pathological 'conditions' impacting fetus/child. But equally, I suggest that we remember to do so in conditions of mediation, involving the 'palpable integration' of media practices 'into our daily lives' (Silverstone, 1999, p. 3).

7 Perinatality and the digital

Cautious optimism

In the preceding chapters, I drew upon findings from online case studies and face-to-face research with women in the context of their everyday lives, trying to grasp the role of media technologies, particularly digital technologies, and environments in the context of what the perinatal has meant for them. My core argument in this book has been that we cannot make sense of or support perinatality in Western societies today, entirely independently of media and communication technologies. The perinatal ideal – my main framework and the conceptual core of the book which returned time and again throughout this work – relied fundamentally on the twin frameworks of mediation and intensive mothering, considering media and communication technologies as inseparable from the ideology of mothering intensively. I conceptualised the perinatal ideal, as an ideology, quite like intensive mothering – an individualising, responsibilising, morally weighted set of conditions, tied fundamentally to the logics of contemporary neo-liberal societies, as Chapter 2 suggested. These conditions are tied, as I also noted, to the moralised, biological specificities of perinatality and they derive their specificity from the particular conditions of the perinatal. These particularities derive from the unique rapidity of infant development which occurs in the first year post-birth, the intense, acute and heightened interfaces with policy and practice in infant well-being and healthcare, with ever-increasing technological advancement that parents, but particularly mothers, engage with increasingly.

I move on to discussing my overall claims and findings the empirical work in this book has made. From these I distil and draw out a set of key conclusions as I think through the implications of digital technology for perinatality, drawing upon my findings in this work. I consider the wide divergences in contexts, expectations and experiences of the digital in this case, ultimately making a cautiously optimistic case through a set of recommendations for the role of digital technologies and environments in this context.

Uneven contexts of access and use

One of the first aspects to note, across my findings, is that not all mothers were online; those that were online were enormously diverse in terms of degrees and nature of access, the expectations they held of online spaces and the practices and literacies which were displayed. This is of course not new information, but at a time when there is significant hope around digital health and 'getting everyone online', the real picture is far more complex and will continue to be so, for there will always be unevenness in all of the above. As findings have also shown, simply being online or simply being in a position to access spaces is not a magic solution to anything. This is partly, as chapters 3 and 4 showed, because of the wide-ranging unevenness in the content available and discourses circulating and being accessed in formal as well as informal arenas. But also, as chapters 5 and 6 demonstrated, this is due to a range of structural pressures which blend online and offline spaces, which mothers will be working within and against, to widely varying degrees. A few conclusions in this strand follow.

The role of offline support networks is complex and should not always be assumed to be supportive

Critical to note is the often spoken-about contextual factor of offline support networks, often female support networks, which, as my findings in chapters 5 and 6 have revealed, paint a less straightforward picture than is expected. In many cases, mothers reported that they did not 'need' to go online, for there were large familial support networks offline. As I have elucidated elsewhere and also as I do below, large offline support networks do not necessarily equate to solely positive outcomes for women, and these networks are often mixed in terms of the degrees of support and sometimes surveillance they seem to provide. In some cases, for instance, for Adela – a second-generation immigrant with very strong relationships with her mother and sister – these offline networks work so wonderfully that she says that she never felt the need to seek out either information or sociality online. However, for Antonia, who had had a very difficult and traumatic experience with childbirth, she says she had "just family supporting, and talked with some friends" – when later it emerges that these networks did not offer her all of what she needed to cope rather than being fulfilling enough for her to not have needed to fill any gaps.

This might prompt us to paint a black and white picture, with the offline and online in separate categories, where offline gaps necessitate online ventures and where the two do not mix or merge. But predictably, there was complexity rather than any picture as straightforward as this. Many who did not go online in search of information or peer support, and who did indeed have large networks on the ground, felt misunderstood and surveilled by these very networks, even when they were, on occasion, supportive. Many who felt this way and found the resources and capital to be able to access online spaces and networks, felt able to escape in ways more than one the large support networks one often hears about framed as a resource. On the ground, support networks sometimes worked as resources, sometimes as restraints, often falling somewhere in between and they shaped and were, in turn, shaped by mothers' experiences online. Online support networks, for instance, People Nearby Applications or summer picnics organised through breastfeeding support groups, often go offline and become part of existing or new offline support networks with their own sets of structural constraints and exclusions.

Interpersonal ties in the perinatal are shaped by online experiences and short-lived online ties are often affectively significant

My findings in Chapter 5 also presented evidence of significant complexities and relative significance in emotional terms of short-lived social ties in digitally mediated perinatal connections. What goes on within these ties online does not stay online, and seeps into mothers' childcare practices, self-perceptions, sense of feeling well and coping with the demands of perinatality. Also, material and emotional roles of traditionally held-to-be-important offline support networks of mothers are often renegotiated, repositioned and even bypassed through online ties. This all takes myriad forms, resulting in a wide spectrum of outcomes and emerging out of widely divergent familial and wider interpersonal contexts offline. Findings in Chapter 6, although more broadly also in Chapter 4, go to show that discourses of support and celebration of good mothering equally function also as discourses of responsibilisation, where supportive resources and rhetoric in contexts of peer support might appear to ease, but might actually maintain the conditions for responsibilising mothers.

Intersectional experiences within easy-to-form groupings of perinatal mothers remind us not to reduce digital access, literacies and practices to individual narratives of success or failure

Women's coping strategies and resilience to such a wide array of cross-cutting rhetoric in conditions of the perinatal ideal are and will continue to be divergent. Some like Nasreen or Raagini reported very high levels of offline social support, high amounts of confidence in their own professional roles and positioned everything perinatal as a question of 'choice' and control. Nasreen confidently spoke of hypnobirthing communities online and her determination to avoid 'a messy birth', and Raagini reported very detailed and organised research online to prepare for birth:

RAAGINI: But I pulled on ... I spent a lot of time on my phone actually. So on the internet looking for people whom ... There's one lady I'd met through ... So I called my midwife in. I was like, do I need to change my birth plan? Do I need to not go for a home birth? I looked online, I looked whether I should be going to a physio or an osteopath or a, you know, kind of ... I called ... One lady I met through the first mum's group kind of they have this little ... I don't know whether it's everywhere but in Hertfordshire you get all mums called to like these four classes and stuff. So I'd met one lady who she deals with family fitness,

> so post foetal fitness. So I called her in as like I need help. So I just pulled on everything and she recommended a physio and it's ... So those were my sources of help.

Raagini's significant confidence and high levels of resilience and literacy contrast starkly to, for instance, Ollee's, whose circumstances of isolation, severity of experiences and emotional struggles, makes it impossible for her to even consider engaging – even speaking to me about her difficulties seems too much for her. As she says:

> I looked on-line to see if I could see any groups, I didn't join any though, I didn't join any. Because I thought have I got PND, I thought that to start with, when I didn't pick her up. And I thought, no, I'll be alright tomorrow, I'll be alright in a few days, but I wasn't. Just feeling ... I just felt really down, didn't want to burden anybody with it, just kept it to myself.

Nasreen and Raagini's experiences with perinatality show practices of questioning discourses, resisting pressures, seeking out online resources such as hypnobirthing tapes from Western natural birthing cultures and blending these with their mothers' advice and counsel on many matters, or meaningful objects from cultures of origin such as the Flower of Fatimah as Nasreen spoke of, carrying these into their experiences of the perinatal. Both showed great resilience and strength, and yet, it is important that we do not read their practices and (digital) literacies and resilience as narratives to be explained at the level of the individual alone. Unlike many other migrant mothers, they came from varying positions of privilege and had a wide range of resources at their disposal. As Gedalof (2009) suggests:

> the question is not only how migrant mothers are constrained by pre-existing structures in their agency, but also, how can we understand both structures and agents of belonging as messy and dynamic entanglements of constraint and enablement, being and becoming, movement and inhabitance.
>
> (p. 88)

This draws attention, amongst other things, to real, lived intersectionality across any potential category we might construct for the perinatal, for instance, 'migrant mothers'.

Many mothers are not online, many who are online appear to seek information only and not support, and telephony continues to be significant

The next strand of critical issues which underlie all the optimistic findings reported in this work is of course the long-standing question of access and digital health. My interviews with migrant mothers, especially those from lower socio-economic backgrounds, showed many accounts of isolation throughout the perinatal period, despite being surrounded by a larger extended family (and often, precisely, due to being surrounded by a larger, extended family by whom many felt surveilled and monitored). Many were entirely offline and often dependent on their husbands to top-up phone calling cards to call sympathetic relatives on a different continent. Evidence from race studies and healthcare shows that ethnic minority migrant mothers face increased postnatal mental health risks (Almeida et al., 2016; Latif, 2014) and migrant mothers struggle particularly with cultural taboos around mental ill-health (NELSHA, 2003).[1] A few studies have investigated in particular the maternal mental health issues faced by migrant mothers (c.f. Almond & Lathlean, 2011; Babatunde & Moreno-Leguizamon, 2012; Edge, 2007a, 2007b; Onozawa et al., 2003). But, as the Race Inequality Commission identifies (2014), there is currently a "knowledge gap regarding the impact of cultural factors on maternal mental disorders" (p. 6), and that existing structures are geared very closely towards Western women and a range of linguistic and cultural barriers stand in the way of migrant mothers finding adequate amounts of postnatal mental health support. For Leticia, a newly arrived migrant mother, with severe experiences of trauma, including child loss in her country of origin, the disconnection, both on and offline, was stark in the face of a sense of feeling overwhelmed with everything that was going on as she arrived in the U.K. As she pointed out to me:

> I wasn't very informed, and also didn't have my chapters. So it was more of ... I'm bothered about getting my papers sorted and I wasn't very aware of all these things I could do to find out information about being pregnant. I also have the African perception in my head where you get pregnant, you go hospital, you get your injection, you give birth and that's it. There's nothing like learning, or reading books, or even going into classes; that things was all new to me.

Leticia's sense of not needing online connections or information links to a stark sense of isolation and feeling overwhelmed in a new country with a significant set of cultural differences to overcome. Many like Nritya or Jemima spoke of using the online very little, for information rather than connection, and some like Rumia emphasised the nature of information found online as necessarily 'not very scientific', emphasising the pursuit of information far more over connection. As noted previously, we cannot extrapolate from this group to conclude that they somehow did not 'need' online ties or sources of support or that their offline networks were always enough or fully satisfactory, because that is not the case in reality. Amongst this group of mothers, who had an information-only rather than connection-based approach to and expectations of online spaces, apps emerge to be significant. Neeta spoke of how apps helped both her and her partner.

Vanini, who did not venture online at all, spoke of the importance to her, almost as a daily ritual, of pregnancy progression apps to keep worries in check. Hema articulates this in her use of an app to cope with low-level worrying about her pregnancy and its progress:

> HEMA: That was a lot of you know, week by week when they tell you how your baby is doing and how your baby is growing, a lot of that. I had one or two books that I bought which I used for information as well.

Following this example, I found consistently lower levels of Internet use, and hence far lower levels of being able to benefit from the many instances of positive and supportive uses of the Internet, keeping in mind of course the many darker, and less than supportive aspects of practices unfolding in these spaces, as discussed in preceding chapters. Harini spoke of significant isolation and of venturing online to find information – but what became significant for her in the end was audio calls and mobile telephony – serving on the one hand to connect her to one or two key relatives, but arguably disconnecting her from a potentially wider network of support, albeit, as we have seen, uneven in nature.

> HARINI: I used to see online, you know, that apps and everything they send you message every week about what's going on with the baby, how growing and I used to do a lot of online search. What to eat, what not to eat, things like that, so. I've got few friends, but all went to work and a bit busy, so we used to talk but not that much. You know how life here is. … We talk through our phones and Skype and things like that.

A heavy use of Internet telephony to connect with families, a larger reliance on in-person services (themselves under pressure in the U.K.) at children's centres and low use of online fora for information or support seeking came up frequently in conversations with mothers from migrant backgrounds who were also socio-economically disadvantaged. In general, amongst this group of mothers, there seemed to be a greater focus on information seeking from the Internet as opposed to support-seeking or venturing into the more social dimensions of online spaces. Having said that, as Chapter 5 demonstrated, some then went on to use this information for broader social purposes within offline networks, and for the vast majority, 'information' about the perinatal was more often than not laden with meaning and affective power under conditions of the perinatal ideal.

Keeping in mind such a wide diversity of contexts of access, use, practices, the nature and severity of perinatal difficulties and even resilience, it is critical thus that high expectations around potential contributions from digital in maternal well-being do not bypass these issues, and can ask critical questions about how the digital can aid inclusive maternal well-being in this context around wider NHS ambitions of delivering culturally competent care.

The case for optimism

I have argued in this book that across a variety of online spaces, extending to the spilling over of such spaces into the offline, there is often great vitality and agency in the support or peers at all hours of struggle in the perinatal period. Particularly, as findings showed in Chapter 4 for instance, the amity extended to mothers to reject and oppose perceived-to-be oppressive advice and technocratic labour cultures is significant. These have remarkably positive and even empowering roles to play, particularly in moments of difficulty and despair where offline support networks. In this section, I report from findings which support the case for positive, even emancipatory uses of digital technologies and interfaces in the perinatal period, covering the long-standing priorities of information seeking, solidarity and support, and also the sense of accessibility and immediacy around the digital that arose from my findings.

Online spaces offer valuable information and support for struggling mothers

Research has evidenced substantially now that women value information and emotional support on well-being related issues in the perinatal period, from accessible, even lay experts online, bypassing or complementing formal sources of information (McKeever & McKeever, 2017; Prescott & Mackie, 2017; Slomian et al, 2017). More generally, women have been evidenced to be using the Internet for health information seeking more than men (Bauman et al., 2017; Myrick & Willoughby, 2017), with good strategies of information seeking online defined as a key health literacy goal (Nutbeam et al., 2017). Online and offline data demonstrated in this work too that women who had access to the Internet valued the sense of agency and initiative that came through self-directed information seeking, often over and above other informal and formal sources of information, and most critically, in terms of bypassing waiting periods to be able to access healthcare professionals, offline or even telephone helplines the morning after a difficult night. While some spoke of turning to formal organisations and their websites in order to find information, many spoke of lurking on or sometimes contributing to discussion forums built to support women perinatally, and run and managed entirely through an online network of peers (as opposed to formally set-up e-health initiatives). For many women, these sources took the place of information handed out at GP surgeries or even through informal face-to-face networks. For some, this becomes particularly pronounced when speaking of specific stages in the perinatal, as women turn to the online world to look for quick answers at all hours of the night, often reporting searching through the advanced search functions of online forums to find discussions in the past which had seen women ask similar questions online. This has value in the context of pressured

NHS services filling in gaps where a woman might have to be waiting to find information she needs and equally, has value in terms of emotional peer-to-peer support (see also Cline & Haynes, 2001). The online appeared to the most easily accessed realm of information, often even sought as a reflex action on the go from smartphones. In each case where a woman spoke of finding information online, these became the most pronounced for questions around infant feeding, infant sleep, baby weaning and postnatal anxiety.

Many online spaces offer open up genuine online and offline avenues for perinatal mothers, for connection, resistance and agency

A key component of this is also the seeking of solidarity and peer support. I note here that most specifically in discussions online of childbirth and birth choices, I found the notion of solidarity and friendliness in the context of the digital perinatal to sit in the context of a longer history of feminist agency within the midwife-led natural birth movement (Kitzinger, 2012b), although I follow this up in a later section with important caveats around the very diminishing of that space of solidarity in certain contexts. Online support around perinatal issues mediates offline support systems, and the expectations women have, the rightful demands they are able to make, of healthcare professionals and their partners and families show up as particularly critical in discussions of childbirth and the postnatal period, as evident in the online exchange above.

In addition, women who have used People Nearby Applications (PNAs) such as MUSH, which enable local mothers to connect with each other, show that the establishment of offline connections and meetups through online interfaces is crucial, emotionally and socially, particularly during the isolation of being on maternity leave, away from work, when partners have usually returned to work. This aligns with recent research on PNAs which show how feelings of safety and trust are fostered prior to offline meetings and their potentials in supporting cultural and social capital (Hsiao & Dillahunt, 2017). Elisa says:

> I have a PhD myself and was working in London, till I found myself here at home, and feeling really cut-off, in this small town. My husband is at work all day and it seemed as though the walls were what I had to speak to. I discovered MUSH and I started meeting up with other mothers in the area. The Children's Centres had never told me about anything like this, and I found it so much easier than going for weekly baby groups which were never convenient.

Online bonds seem to become particularly reinforced when they move offline, suggesting potentially the value of using portals such as the above to establish supportive local groups, providing we stay wary of commercial providers and intrusions on personal data. This is also something evidenced in women's accounts of using breastfeeding support groups which have a simultaneous online and offline presence. In many instances, women spoke of pressures and even intrusions from well-meaning but pressure-creating family support systems, where they felt unable to explain themselves, which led them to look for support that was accessible and available online, which in turn moved towards newer offline connections of support. As Monica, a mother who initially struggled to establish breastfeeding, said to me:

> My mother and mother-in-law both were insisting that my daughter was not gaining weight fast enough and the health visitors wouldn't see me because they found her 'fine'. It was when I started exploring the Facebook groups on breastfeeding support and went along to one of their summer picnics that I realized that actually she is okay, and I am doing okay – it helped to see that I wasn't making all the mistakes that my well-meaning relatives were insisting I was making by feeding her myself.

There are key gap-filling roles performed by digital spaces in perinatality

This all points to the critical role of immediacy in terms of finding both information and support and the need for women to speak with other women, online and offline, about the many challenges of the perinatal. The 24/7 nature of the need for information and support for questions that are private, sometimes even embarrassing for some (particularly evident in the case of discussing post-birth intimate issues), women spoke of what I describe as a 'gap-filling' role of digital interfaces and platforms. I use the term to indicate the gap filled between things – sometimes bridging the time gap between an immediate need or query and any potential, formal, offline support; sometimes, bridging the gaps between queries mothers felt able to express when face to face with care providers, and those which felt far too private or far too intimate to be able to disclose in any non-anonymous situation; or sometimes bridging the gap between feeling entirely isolated and alone and being able to muster up the energy to venture outside to an offline group. These key 'in-between' areas were often fruitfully filled through the digital for those who had access and who were regular users.

This gap-filling role was found to occur in at least three ways. First, in the space that falls between being able to ask for support on private, even intimate queries (for instance, when dealing with questions such as conjugal relationships after childbirth, as the woman below says), women spoke of the anonymity, immediacy and the wealth of experience opened up through sharing experiences on online forums and finding the support in the here and the now. As one woman explained in discussing how to soothe an episiotomy immediately post-birth:

> I would never have known that witch hazel and lavender would be of such great comfort post-birth, and the ladies online practically helped me pack my hospital bag. They were also very helpful in thinking about the issues involved with ... you know... returning to stuff with my husband ... after having a baby.

The second key gap-filling role came up in conversations with women who looked back at their experiences of coping with both diagnosed and undiagnosed forms of postnatal depression and anxiety. Many spoke of the convenience and the 'low key'-ness of posting online or even reading up about others' experiences of postnatal emotional difficulties, when they personally found themselves unable to face a large group, or social interactions in offline spaces or unable to cope with both real and perceived stigma around mental health difficulties from family (see also Moore & Ayers, 2017). Livia captures this in her comments:

> When you are not really in a place to put paste on a brush, and are just about able to do the school run and come back home with a colicky baby, with all the groups in the world you might go and sit at, if you can't, you can't can you? I just lurked, and once I saw others were like me, staying in, I started to post, and after a while, of talking (air quotes) to others I felt a bit better and able to drag myself to the real world and try to get you know ... more support there.

The third and more obvious gap-filling role emerged purely as a question of temporality and had to do with the very nature of the perinatal. This included the dynamics of night waking with infants, solitude and isolation in often being the person doing feeds at night while partners slept in preparation for work in the morning, and the unavailability of telephone helplines at that hour which emerged to be important in women reaching out to each other online. Sarah spoke of these spaces as bridging temporal gaps between seeing strong, offline networks and finding emotional support when other (strong) networks were unavailable. She says:

> I had only one friend at the time who'd had children. But then, I made a baby group. And we got six of us in our baby group. It was really quick. And our local, it was like a free place, we'd go there. They did these baby groups. And there was six of us. And we met after. And we still see each other about once a week ... But where you're the only person awake at 3:00 AM with a crying baby, you're not. And yes, so I found them (online spaces) quite useful.

Equally, long waiting periods for offline help in many areas, rushed face-to-face appointments and problems perceived to be too unimportant to merit a visit to healthcare professionals which nonetheless had cumulative impacts on maternal well-being, all seemed to feed into women going online for information, solidarity and support. All these bridging roles filled gaps, I found, between the very real, experiencing of a problem and the accessing of some formal, offline, professional support.

Digitally mediated ties might positively complement rework or reshape existing offline support networks

As Chapter 5 argued, my findings indicated that the challenges to pre-existing offline ties during the perinatal period, themselves down to already-mediated, wider structural issues, led to the increased seeking out of ephemeral but nonetheless affectively impactful weaker tie connections online, some of which moved offline. But equally, discussions about these structural issues impacting interpersonal relationships if offline, strong tie relationships and shaping the materiality of mother's lives offline, including the amount of instrumental and material social support they could access, reshaped for many mothers their expectations of and approaches to these offline, strong tie relationships. Charlotte's account of seeking out local mothers through People Nearby Applications, Moumita and Vanini's gap filling of existing near and far offline familial networks through their agentic use of apps and information seeking or Nasreen's negotiation of her wishes and voices in the context of a gendered relationship dynamic through the use of online information elucidate the often empowering mediating and shaping role of the digital in the context of both new and existing perinatal interpersonal ties.

The case for caution

In what follows, I move now to the darker sides of discourses and interfaces in digital environments, which is particularly important, I suggest, in contexts of easily resorted-to techno-euphoria when it comes to perceiving the digital as a box out there, promising solutions to problems. Findings in previous chapters have outlined that the perinatal is heavily moralised in conditions of intensive mothering.

Counter-discourses are complex, many inclusions produce exclusions and vice versa

This book has presented findings on a range of exclusions and cliques, new lines of marginalisation which might be reproduced or opened up in online spaces or as online ties move offline. But these are also the very ties and spaces which open up potentials for resistance and counter-discourses – not just theoretically, but also counter-discourses circulating in media and culture, and specifically those which might come from organisations that do offer to support maternal depression and anxiety by breaking down the perinatal ideal. But as earlier chapters have elucidated, what appears as inclusive and supportive counter-discourses for one might very well function as a thoroughly exclusive and marginalising discourse for another for the heavy moralising associated with the vast majority of elements in the perinatal. For instance, the Fed is Best movement resists pressures, both perceived and real, to breastfeed. But the movement itself sits against other movements on and offline which aim to encourage and empower women to exclusively breastfeed, which are themselves resistances perhaps against over-medicalised infant feeding practices. The often contrasting and emotionally heavy exchanges, which result at the fringes of these two sets of inclusive (within themselves) pockets of resistance, lead me to suggest that it is not as though spaces for resistance do not exist or open up on/offline on key issues at the heart of the perinatal. They indeed do, and in very many ways, agency, friendship and support features in these pockets of support and resistance. But the perinatal ideal sees conditions where each issue in perinatality is heavily moralised, and hence, what might act as a supportive group practising real resistance to a particular dominant paradigm, and thus, what is an inclusive space for those on the inside, acts also as an exclusive space for those on the outside, with their own discourses to resist. So, indeed there are discourses and counter-discourses, but the raw, often fraught edges and boundaries of these, both on and offline, remind us of how all exclusions produce inclusions and all inclusions might produce exclusions – the cosy 'we' (Phoenix, 2019). This leads me now to discuss the case for caution in approaching the digital in the context of perinatal well-being.

The morally intense nature of some online environments within broader, gendered structures of perinatality necessitate caution in place of assuming that all peer support spaces online are uniform or uniformly useful

Findings in Chapter 4, for instance, provide natural birthing discussions as a useful case to study this. There have been pendulum shifts in our mediated frameworks of reference in speaking about the perinatal and perinatal maternal bodies. On the one hand, this framework represents the laudable premises of natural birthing which involved a justifiable questioning of white-coated obstetrics. On the other hand, despite the emphasis in this discourse on maternal choice, there are boundaries and limits placed on what maternal behaviour will be supported, what will merely be tolerated and what is most unwelcome.

So, we need to pay attention to questions of exclusion and silencing on online platforms (see also Miller et al., 2007, Lee, 2008 and Faircloth, 2010, writing on discourses of exclusion when mothering does not fit the norms of ideal/superior practices of feeding or birthing). In previous chapters I have explored some of these issues as being linked to an environment of intensive mothering (Hays, 1998) and demonstrated, with empirical evidence, how women who have had difficult or traumatic birth experiences have felt silenced online. I have argued that in parallel to the real sense of agency and alliance in the genuine victories of the natural birth movement, contemporary practices of intensive birth preparation and the digital curation and maintenance of an almost euphoric and uniformly positive birth that even prohibits the use of the word 'pain' in certain online spaces serves to both silence and concern women, who then go on to feel as though they are to blame for any birth experience which is less than positive. Both these discourses – one emancipatory and empowering, and the other, intensively self-responsible and exclusionary – appeared in both online and offline encounters, and often in social ties which spanned both digital and offline spaces seamlessly, for instance, in friendship networks. Charmaine grasped the latter, when she spoke to me of how her birth story – which involved the use of the word 'pain' – was eliminated from an online space populated by a group of women she had grown to trust and consider to be her friends:

> I felt quite let down ... within that community of people who want to birth naturally, you know, I would welcome more people saying it really hurt. There are techniques you can adopt to cope with it, but be prepared, it's really hard.

As I have noted in Chapter 3, from my analysis of online fora and the rules put in place around language and permissible and not permissible birth debriefs, silences and exclusions are as critical to note as supportive rapports and inclusivity. Many women, in the course of fieldwork, noted to me that, for instance, verbalising pain, including even swearing profusely in labour, gave pain a recognition, a legitimacy and that helped them in recognising the hard work that labour truly is. And yet, in placing strict guidelines on the terminology that is permitted on many online spaces on birthing, some voices are shut down in a broader environment of intensive mothering where the mother must sacrifice and bear (see also Mack, 2016, for an excellent analysis of masochism and birthing videos) and even transcend all pain for the sake of her child. As my research showed, on a Facebook group, a woman who had a traumatic birth came looking for support but was attacked by other group members for sharing her account. It is important that we recognise that online spaces are far from simple, and speak to, feed out of and feed into wider discourses around parenting, motherhood, responsibility and self-management.

Pervasive discourses of individualisation responsibilise mothers over and again

Whether one looks at the rhetoric circulating within online spaces around perinatality or around formal and official literature and resources mothers are surrounded by or by the structural changes and shifts which perinatal support for mothers is undergoing as we speak, a discourse of pervasive individualisation runs clear and strong throughout. I looked at this in detail in terms of analysing rhetoric on childbirth support groups online in Chapter 4, where birthing, particularly *good* birthing, was very much positioned as an individual achievement, an individual responsibility and hence, an individual failure when things went wrong. This permeated women's abilities to speak about their births, concealing or toning down speech about good experiences and feeling and experiencing isolation and prejudice when attempting to speak about difficult experiences. The moral weight of motherhood in neo-liberal societies is rendered particularly visible in the perinatal period, as I posited in Chapter 2. This complicates boundaries between information and communication, as I suggested in Chapter 5, so that all information on perinatal issues, from formal as well as informal sources, is read against and often offered against a backdrop which continues to tie infant to mother, mobilising subtle and not-so-subtle rhetoric of individual women needing to mother intensively. As noted in Chapter 6, this also forms the structures through which affective experiences of difficult emotions, for instance, anxiety and self-doubt (rationalised, understood, framed and treated nearly always at the level of the individual mother) makes its way through on and offline spaces, spilling across objects and materiality.

In women's talk about their own responsibilities to birth well, feed well, wean well, whether speaking about discussions online or peer support online or about the broader spectrum of circulating ideas derived from a range of formal, familial and wider sources, maternal instinct is valued highly. As I demonstrated in chapters 3 and 4, this sits between two positions on each side of the same coin, one, where a recognition of instinct, agency and autonomy marked the victory of agentic, women-led practices in perinatality, rejecting largely male and often over-medicalised stances, and the other, where that very instinct becomes an individual goalpost, achievement and burden, tying mother to child. Chapter 4 demonstrated, for instance, how mothers' instinct is highly valued, which despite historically rightly being a remarkable retort to over-medicalisation of the perinatal, often sees women being supported emphatically within the community to do their utmost best by their children, by refraining from using certain words and by speaking only of positive, joyful experiences. There is a price attached in certain circles, then, of speaking openly about ambiguity or difficulties in relation to birth or infant feeding, for valuable social ties, in which one has already invested emotionally, are significantly at stake.

Likewise, in Chapter 6, I spoke the 'red herring of infant well-being', where I suggested that in digital societies, perinatal anxiety often becomes visible, finds reassurance and is produced and maintained in the form of minute and specific infant well-being related queries and worries, but is essentially rooted in ideals and ideologies surrounding mother blame, where individual women worry about not being good enough mothers, feeding well or consistently enough, weaning too early or too late. These, like birthing-related issues, as discussed in Chapter 4, see various perinatal specificities, for instance, around the mode of birth and the use or rejection of pain relief become moralised indicators of how 'well' a mother is perceived or perceives herself to have done in every rapid-onset stage of the perinatal.

I also noted, in Chapter 6, but more broadly that peer support itself might over-responsibilise twice over. At its broadest level, as state support recedes for health services, generating enormous pressure on healthcare professionals and on women who struggle to find face-to-face support, online peer support might appear as a miracle solution. Yet, it creates a burden of self-support and peer support on individuals and communities struggling with perinatal anxiety as state support recedes. Equally, even within the discourses of support, notwithstanding cliques of inclusivity and exclusivity, as discussed in Chapter 4, the rhetoric of support itself might often reinforce pressures to be a 'great mother', which subtly and often even unintentionally serves to burden and responsibilise, as noted in Chapter 6. In either case, it seems clear that the onus of seeking and finding (the right kind) of online support is increasingly on the anxious mother herself, at the level of the individual. So, it is worthwhile considering with care the broader and pervasive forces of intensive mothering, within national contexts of receding state support, and the burden of support on communities where many are suffering equally, when we set out to consider the expectations we place of online peer support.

Mothers, bodies and perinatality are all increasingly data and increasingly dataveilled

Worthy enormously of further study, is increasing dataveillance and self-monitoring through the latest devices and monitoring which invite new avenues of comparing, tracking, monitoring, surveilling, managing and find relief and comfort geared around the specificities of infant well-being, but all maintaining conditions of intense individual burden on women under broader conditions of intensive mothering (Barassi, 2017). Research around perinatality and the digital must pay attention to the critical conversations arising around datafication (Van Dijck, 2014), quantification and the digital in the context of health and well-being facing digital interfaces (c.f. Lupton, 2016). The most personal, private and intimate aspects of female bodies can be quantified through the daily monitoring of bodily temperatures, fluids, emotional states and then fed into a broader pool of data, which will apparently improve insights and predictions of fertility and menstruation. Commercial intrusions are key here. Algorithmic targeting of adverts on social networking spaces, for instance, increasingly invite women to chart their fertility data throughout the month, aiming, seemingly, to put women 'in control' of their bodies. This extends beyond the charting of monthly periods on a calendar application and extends to the mapping and submitting to an unknown bank of data out there, a variety of other details, including ovulation, diet, mood, exercise etc. As scholars succinctly argue (Choe et al., 2014; Lupton, 2016; Mol, 2000, amongst others), these applications encourage women to live in a permanent state of anxiety and close monitoring of their own bodies, perhaps even increasing anxiety rather than relieving it. I found in my conversations with women that they presented conflicting discourses around these invitations to self-monitor and self-regulate in the context of fertility and conception. Often these were described as being "fully in control of knowing when I am due on ... and then when I'm going to ovulate, so really convenient and keeping me in the loop about my own body" – and also, by the same participant when trying unsuccessfully to conceive, "my temperature did not rise the way it was meant to, and this probably means another month and I have not conceived". These contrasting repertoires of feeling apparently in control, but then having the sense of control dependent entirely on scrutinising one's body for symptoms and going through the highs and lows of expectations and disappointment, raise critical questions around the potential emotional implications of these many fertility apps and the rhetoric of control and agency they seem to present. This datafication of fertility and its consequences in critical digital health studies (c.f. Lupton, 2017) also feeds into neo-liberal discourses of individualisation and self-management.

Equally deserving of careful attention is the second critical issue around this phenomenon of datafied fertility which arise around women's everyday interactions with algorithms (see also Bucher, 2017) online, as targeted advertizing leads to the commercial encroachment by these very fertility and conception apps, interrupting and punctuating online activity. The commodification and datafication of fertility, leading to algorithmic intrusions of women's browsing experiences and indeed their lived, everyday lives thus beckon critical investigation. The third issue, as many note in terms of health data (c.f. Lupton, 2016; Meißner, 2016), is the ambiguity and lack of transparency of fertility data from the moment data is submitted into an ethereal pool of data – what happens to it? What contextualises it? What kind of critical data literacies are necessitated as women interface with these apps? While my project did not find the space to incorporate such issues, the use of apps and the surfacing of these even during our interviews draws attention to the increasingly pervasive nature of such practices and demands attention in future research.

Cautious optimism: representations, connections, intrusions

The findings discussed above focuses us on issues arising at the intersections of digital societies and the perinatal, to draw attention to the contradictions, tensions and juxtaposition of discourse. This beckons both optimism and caution, distancing itself from euphoric rhetoric around the potentials of the digital, while making a case for carving space for mothers, especially in the vulnerable periods of the perinatal. I locate this work against the long history of theorisation of mediated communication, which considers how the media, in this case, digital media, are inseparable from societal processes and institutions, making this claim not in a celebratory or cynical note, but rather emphasising the transformations of practices, processes and institutions in complex ways, with the arrival of various waves of media and communication technologies. Within the context of this mediated framework, we have time and again seen rich, in-depth qualitative work, although not solely so, speaking about the social shaping of technology (Mackenzie & Wajcman, 1999) and the appropriation of digital interfaces (c.f. Woolgar, 2002). We have arrived at key concepts across overlapping waves of the digital (Fuchs et al., 2010). These include a theorisation of interpersonal relationships in the digital age (c.f. Baym, 2015; c.f. Madianou & Miller, 2012), conceptualisations of social capital online (c.f. Ellison et al., 2008), theorisation of media and digital literacies, including also data and algorithm literacies (c.f. Livingstone, 2008), critical and contextual approaches to studying both risks and opportunities associated with Internet use in specific socio-cultural groups (c.f. Livingstone, 2013), the location of digital interfaces and technologies in everyday life (c.f. Bakardjieva, 2005; Bucher, 2017) and the implications arising at the intersect of the newest wave of algorithmic, datafied interfaces (Van Dijck, 2014) and critical digital well-being (c.f. Lupton, 2016, 2017). Across all of these strands of work and more, a mediated communicative framework has consistently drawn us away from approaching technology through lenses of either unqualified hope or hype, away from panic and euphoria alike.

Earlier in this book, I suggested in Chapter 2 that the transformations as we live in digital societies mean that the perinatal is being shaped as we speak in at least three cross-cutting ways, all of which are morphing through successive waves of mediation. The first I suggested was the ever-important question of *representations*, drawing our attention to newer visual cultures of self-representation, aided by algorithmic monitoring, highlighting and silencing. The second I suggested was interpersonal *connections* and the wide array of practices, both empowering and exclusionary, which are at play, blending online and offline spaces of the perinatal. The third, which this book has been unable to look into but which is increasingly worthy of critical scrutiny, is the question of *intrusions*, whereby perinatality, bodies and emotions are all increasingly data. In this book, I partly took up what Lupton sets out above in terms of examining what exactly is going on at the intersections of the perinatal and the digital. My findings hovered around examining what is going on, but I aim to use the conclusions and findings developed here to move towards setting out some recommendations for perinatality in the digital in the broader U.K. context in what follows.

In the sections below, I think about maternal emotional well-being in the perinatal period and contemplate the potential roles digital technologies might play in the process. To do so, it is important that we locate this in the particular public policy contexts of the U.K., within which maternal well-being in early years is framed and approached. I argue that nesting it within service provision for infants and very young children, overlapping with austerity measures and public funding cuts, prevents a distinct space emerging for maternal well-being.

Throughout this book ran an emphasis – which the subtitle of the book partly reflects – on pressures and struggles of the perinatal, drawing our attention to discourses, rhetoric, practices and logics of what underpins, produces and maintains some of these difficulties and struggles for mothers. I produced a set of findings around the roles and potentials of new technologies in perinatality across the chapters of this work. It is worth articulating at the outset why I selected to group the kinds of mediated experiences I spoke in this book, and why my conclusions move me towards speaking specifically now to the notion of maternal *well-being* in the perinatal period, which is the note on which this book ends. This book is not one that has spoken psychologically or bio-medically to the measures and outcomes of well-being as it is understood in these fields after all, but focused instead on the mediated, sociological structures, rhetoric, pressures and struggles which punctuate early motherhood for many, locating a focus on the difficult and the turbulent, if one will, from the outset. The four substantial strands to this book – birthing discourses in representations, similar discourses in talk, interpersonal ties in the perinatal period and perinatal anxieties – all revolved around issues to do with pregnancy, birth and the immediate post-birth postnatal period, and they all related to discourses of and around the *perinatal*. The connection to well-being relates to the arguments made in Chapter 6, i.e. the struggles, pressures and deeply gendered ideals and rhetoric, which come across throughout the book, remind us that we need to approach any conversations on maternal well-being, including struggles with emotional difficulties, in a mediated, sociological framework and not a solely individual clinical one.

So, parts of this book interrogated the nuances of digitally mediated birthing rhetoric and queried the potential outcomes of selective validation and silencing of birthing narratives. Other parts considered the nuances of mediated interpersonal ties in the perinatal period and considered the mediation of perinatal anxiety – to be understood not in an individual, pathological sense (alone). These all provide the backdrops and contexts, I suggest, against which emotional well-being difficulties in the perinatal might be fruitfully understood. Rather than the rest of this book and the recommendations it puts forward being *about* the measures and outcomes of perinatal well-being at all, it becomes then about the mediated *contexts* of perinatal struggles and pressures, within which we might begin to unpack, amongst a variety of other things, the ways in which the digital can and cannot potentially support maternal perinatal well-being. The concept of maternal *well-being* is of increasing use in public policy discourse, bio-medical literature and indeed sits within a broader history of interest in the *sociology* of well-being (c.d. Carlisle et al., 2009; Carlisle & Hanlon, 2008). The sociology of well-being links the individual to the societal, including the institutional, and offers an inroad into looking at maternal well-being in line with the extensively developed scholarship around maternal subjectivities, identities and agency, which I delved into in Chapter 2. My use of the term *well-being* itself in this context, thus, steps away from its psychological or biomedical underpinnings and looks more broadly into anxieties, ideals and relationships during the critical perinatal period – and provides a mediated account of the communicative contexts of the perinatal, within which, I suggest, we understand the increasingly discussed and popular notions of perinatal anxiety and related emotional difficulties. This ran through this book with its focus on pressures and struggles of early motherhood.

A space for the perinatal in digital well-being

As Lupton notes rightly, "the movement of digital health technologies into new arenas such as ... prenatal and postnatal care for and surveillance of new mothers and their infants requires further research" (Lupton, 2014, p. 1355). This invites an investigation of the contextualised practices arising around the use of digital interfaces and platforms for perinatal health and well-being, whether these are community/peer led and supported or more formal interventions. This also invites an everyday life engagement with ongoing critiques around intrusive interfaces (Mollen & Dhaenens, 2018) and datafication (c.f. Van Dijck, 2014), and the ways in which women are invited, often algorithmically, by commercial organisations or even by e-health initiatives to monitor and quantify their biological data (c.f. Lupton, 2017). So we need to pay attention to brighter and darker sides of technology and its use in the perinatal, some of which have appeared in the findings presented in this book, and in the recommendations it produces. A critical body of research on e-health, m-health and the role of digital technologies in health and well-being has by now accumulated and been reviewed excellently in the literature (Hardey, 2010; Lupton, 2014), including investigations of the challenges and roadblocks in these contexts (Greenhalgh & Keen, 2014; Harvey, 2016). Distilling the findings of all the work that falls under these areas, including what Lupton usefully terms *critical digital health studies* (2014), is not possible to do in this chapter, and in what follows, I draw attention to two kinds of research, both of which are of significance, I suggest, to the area under investigation here, but each of which draws upon somewhat different priorities. On the one hand, there is rich literature, operating largely, although not solely, within a social scientific approach, which has produced critical insights on women's use of online fora for information seeking, solidarity, support and empathy, in all matters concerning the perinatal, extending from infant feeding to child health in general and from pregnancy and conception to postnatal depression (Chalklen & Anderson, 2017; Cheresheva, 2015; Madge and O'Connor, 2006; O'Connor and Madge, 2004; Schaan & Melzer, 2015). This work has partly focused on maternal discourses online and has often read these through the critical lens of performances of intensive mothering, and the production of 'good' and 'bad' mothers, for example (c.f. Pedersen & Smithson, 2013). On the other hand, another branch of work, not directly related to digital health and well-being per se but producing consistently rich and critical findings around the mediation of motherhood, has emerged from a long line of research looking at the pressures on mothering in austerity, and in the context of public funding cuts, and the intersections of media, technologies, neo-liberal policies and motherhood (c.f. Bochantin et al., 2010; Douglas & Michaels, 2005; O'Brien Hallstein, 2011; Moravec, 2011; O'Donohoe et al., 2013; Tyler, 2009). These take into account political-economic and cultural contexts within which maternal subjectivities are produced and maintained. While these two branches of work – one at the intersections of social science disciplines and information and communication technologies in the context of health, and the other, taking critical-cultural studies and political-economic approaches into the discourses around motherhood in austere and neo-liberal times – may seem disconnected, both literatures have the best interests of mothers at their core, arguing from a variety of critical positions for more progressive technological, societal and cultural outcomes for women.

In the context of England and the National Health Service, these two literatures speak closely to each other, specifically because austerity and public funding cuts to support systems and services for mothers (in the context of austerity and budget cuts more widely, for public institutions) create societal, political and cultural conditions that draw together both these strands of work. The public policy context around perinatality and the digital is particularly relevant here, and this is a complex terrain with a long history of policies, some around mental health, some around maternal well-being and an entire body of material around digital strategies and policies within the National Health Services. A few points are critical to note. The first relates to a gap in provision for mothers in the critical perinatal period. Taking the instance of mental health alone, it is widely evidenced that Health Visiting services are struggling in England (*The Guardian*, 2018) owing to public funding cuts and 3% NHS trusts have a concrete postnatal mental health strategy in place (BBC, 2016). The Health Visitor Implementation Plan (2011–2015) notes that while primary care initiatives, for instance, investment in health visitors and the introduction of six-week screenings for mothers to identify maternal emotional well-being issues, have been useful, a significant amount of unfulfilled need remains simply because Health Visiting capacities are continuing to struggle. The Royal College of Midwives acknowledge this as the outcome of an uneven and inadequate system (Royal College of Midwives, 2014) of postcode lottery for support allocation locally – a system which has been found 'unacceptable' by NHS England (2016). Over the course of the last decade, such changes have been noticed and noted widely across the nursing, health visiting and midwifery sector. It was noted in 2013 that half of English regions had cut their spending on maternity services (TPA, 2013). Maternity Action concluded in its 2014 report that:

> Since 2010, the Government has made a series of cuts to benefits and statutory payments targeted at or available to pregnant women and parents of children aged up to 12 months ... (and) these cuts are exacerbating the high rate of poverty among new families.
>
> (MA, 2014)

And yet, recently, there has been cause for renewed optimism. An NHS Review (2017) noted that in March 2015, the Government announced that £1.25 billion would be spent on mental health services for children and new mothers over the next parliament, with £75 million over five years earmarked for providing the "right care to more women who experience mental ill health during the perinatal or antenatal period" (NHS, p. 6). The NHS then announced, as this book was written up, that:

> as part of the £365 million investment in perinatal mental health services, a second wave of NHS England funding means that across 2018/19 £23 million will go to 35 sites around the country to ensure improved access to treatment and better outcomes for women and families.[2]

But, as the BMA noted in 2018 in its Lost in Transit report, "Despite the high prevalence rate of perinatal mental health problems, the provision of perinatal services has been poor" *and that despite* "welcome commitments have been made to increased funding for mental health services ... there are concerns, however, that this is not reaching frontline services" (BMA, 2018, p. 1).

The second aspect to note in the policy context is that the NHS has long had a relationship with the digital, and sometimes, like in many other areas of public life, these discourses aligning with techno-euphoric stances. As Harvey notes poignantly, "it has been challenging to judge the impact of digital healthcare solutions in England despite powerful rhetoric regarding its transformational potential; society, it appears, is unconvinced of this potential" (2016, p. 537). Koteyko et al. (2015), in their analysis of discourses around social networking sites and health, also note the same celebratory undertones around potentials "while marginalising the factors that influence users' online and offline practices and contexts" (p. 468). Indeed, at the time of writing this chapter, the term 'trailblazing' is employed to the recent proposition of testing digital services for mental health in seven areas of England, for instance, including the trial of innovative apps to improve access to care and patient records. The Five Year Forward View for Mental Health predicts, optimistically:

> that digital technology is going to play a crucial role in developing mental health services and the Wachter Review highlights the importance of a digital NHS system that would improve the quality of healthcare and lower costs at the same time.

These are ambitious expectations, and as I conclude in what follows, there is a case for (cautious) optimism and ambitions around the potentials of the digital in the case of the perinatal. But, as Harvey (2016) notes, these need to be approached realistically. But even setting aside the issues around techno-optimism and techno-euphoria, the maternal, especially the perinatal, seems noticeably missing as a concrete and distinct component of these plans, albeit recognised occasionally within digital child health discourse. For instance, it is acknowledged that:

> costs of perinatal mental ill health are estimated at £8.1 billion for each annual birth cohort, or almost £10,000 per birth. Yet fewer than 15 per cent of localities provide effective specialist community perinatal services for women with severe or complex conditions, and more than 40 per cent provide no service at all.
>
> (IMHF, p. 6)

And yet a coherent maternal digital well-being policy seems elusive. While, for instance, the proliferation of a range of useful apps is worthy of noting, might women do well with a suite of apps developed by non-commercial, not intrusive entities which foregrounds specifically maternal well-being as a distinct category? While a variety of apps under a variety of categories, including mental health, may well apply, something tailored and targeted for perinatality and mothers might seem conspicuous by absence. Of course, any gaps in terms of a space for maternal well-being in the digital ambitions also link to gaps in offline provision. So what follows, now considers the findings presented in this book by asking – is there merit in high degrees of optimism around digital solutions in this context? How much do we know about how mothers' online practices link to their offline lives? Does maternal well-being stand to benefit from a more distinct space in the NHS digital strategy? How can challenges be met through constructive, supportive and fair use of the Internet by a variety of sectors?

Locating the perinatal in digital well-being

This work leads me to conclude that there is a great need, as always with all things digital, to remove oneself from both euphoria and panic and to balance optimism and caution. On the whole, I suggest a cautiously optimistic position with regard to engaging digital technologies in supporting mothers perinatally. Such a position entails, I suggest, a careful eye on the myriad systemic, structural, political and economic constraints within and against which such technologies are always embedded, as well as noting the creative, agentic and fruitful pathways taken up with such interfaces, as well as possibilities for supporting individuals and communities and involving institutions which are, and must be resourced to be, involved in regular offline support. To identify a set of next steps and change which might be useful and feasible, it is useful to pay attention to who the key actors are and where mothers are in the process. Key actors might include, for instance, health care services commissioners, healthcare professionals and providers, informal maternity support services, local authorities, Children's Centres, Public Libraries, Voluntary Organisations and specialist charities and industry. Of interest here is the NHS Digital Inclusion Report which aims to "build the capacity of all citizens to access information" and "develop partnerships with the voluntary sector and industry to support digital inclusion". A very brief section on scammers and fake news follows what are very ambitious expectations, I suggest here that paying attention to the messiness of the digital is crucial here, if we are to begin filling gaps in the perinatal through digital 'solutions'.

What can the NHS, as an institution which is subject to funding cuts, or healthcare practitioners with resultant heavy caseloads do when confronted by contextual restraints and structural pressures of the kind this book has spoken about? How might mothers, whilst they continue to struggle against structure multiple times over, be resourced to make the most of opportunities the digital might present in this context? Are there opportunities for countering restraints that might work here? Is it the case that very large-scale, entirely new digital initiatives are sorely needed in this area in keeping with wider optimism around digital health? Or is it the case that more rudimentary steps investigating resources and practices which already exist to begin cross-sector liaisons and partnerships might prove more fruitful, for instance, building partnerships with existing in/semi-formal online communities? Such 'small' steps might necessitate significant attempts to address or at least speak to systemic, structural issues shaping and compounding perinatal difficulties for women. In what follows, I move from these findings to develop suggestions around digital maternal well-being, addressing the National Health Service in the U.K., particularly in the context of its Digital Strategy, and then mothers in the perinatal period. I suggest that a distinct place for maternal digital well-being in the NHS digital strategy would be useful in:

- Distinguishing specific perinatal well-being needs of mothers, recognising cultural differences in approaches to well-being and digital health divides in the U.K.
- Recognising key voices, key trends, gaps and contextual factors in maternal use of technology for mental health and well-being, rejecting techno-euphoria around e-health solutions.

- Building partnerships with existing in/semi-formal online communities where healthcare professional presence would be useful.
- Expanding the current library of mobile apps for well-being to include maternal well-being in a broader context of commercial apps proliferating and constant invitations arriving to self-monitor and hand over one's data.
- Building digital sites to better support mothers, drawing lessons from existing informal, community-led platforms.
- Ensuring continued support for offline support services for which the digital is not a substitute.
- Ensuring that training of offline services includes training on digital well-being.

The NHS frames patients as citizens in its personalised health and care framework 2020 framework of action. By adopting the formulation of the citizen (as opposed to customer or client), the NHS embraces its social and democratic responsibilities in the public sphere, and this ambition underlies its Digital Strategy in terms of policies around data, for instance, as it says, "in the future, it will increasingly be the citizen who determines who has access to their data, with care professionals responding to and respecting their preferences" (NIB, 2014a, p. 22). This ambition of framing patients as citizens is critical, for hopefully it envisages and produces patients as active participants in their own well-being while embracing the institution's responsibilities for competent care provision. Within this framework, there is the ambition and space then to develop a tailored and targeted maternal digital well-being policy, currently lacking – in discursively apparent terms – in its digital plans as it stands at the moment. While of course maternal, indeed parental, and family well-being is linked to children's health and well-being, there needs to be reflection on whether grouping these together does sufficient justice to the individuals involved. A concrete and distinct place for maternal digital well-being, distinct from digital child health (NIB, 2016) in the NHS digital strategy, would go a long way in distinguishing and recognising the specific needs of mothers, as diverse as their contexts are, and developing contextualised and measured solutions which researches and recognises these specificities and differences. Such a strategy would need to be context-sensitive and note much researched issues around access and diversity in cultural approaches to healthcare and health information seeking that characterises maternity in the U.K. As critical communications scholars who stand back from technological determinism, it is imperative to note that technology is not a magic bullet, to be applied, updated, applied, updated, and that will produce finer and better outcomes for mothers in the perinatal context. The suggestions around the carving of space for the maternal in an overall digital strategy, as below, therefore do not arise from a position of approaching digital interfaces and environments as magic bullets, but rather as complex and context-dependent factors which need contextualised research and a balance between techno-euphoric and tech-cynical perspectives.

What might need to be a part of such a stance? First, beginning from where we are would be a good step. A lot is happening in terms of community-led and peer-supported informal networks. I have suggested above that peer support is a complex matter, often support communities are burdened twice over, and that these informal self-help groups cannot be a pathway for state support to retreat. But to begin where we are, the more optimistic and hopeful sides of online support communities might be useful, including Twitter hashtags on postnatal depression support, online parenting forums, chat groups on social networking sites and applications that seem to be enabling mothers to come together. As discussed above in my conclusions, these might mean that a concrete maternal digital well-being strategy would not entail the reinvention of wheels. Much of what exists currently, informally, is community-led and built and, as findings above have shown, the most useful ones seem to be blending online and offline support. Taking full stock of how online peer-led support is making a difference in offline lives, or helping to connect women offline or offering solutions (consider People Nearby Applications like MUSH or infant feeding support group meetings offline, which spread their networks and words online) is one way to begin establishing the real roles played by these, in women's lives perinatally, and the kinds of gaps in provision in the context of funding cuts that these might seem to fill. This needs to bear in mind the load on mothers themselves and emotional labour invested within these peer communities, which I have addressed in Chapter 6.

Next, liaising with these existing provisions, subject of course to appropriate vetting and scrutiny, might be a useful step. This could mean, for instance, the availability of healthcare professionals on some of these spaces, at some times. It could include enabling inter-institution conversations between charities and third sector bodies and the NHS itself, to protect critical digital spaces from commercial encroachment. It would also include ensuring that offline centres of support, for instance, Children's Centres, are fully connected to the strategy and able to guide mothers to useful online avenues. This may also mean that certain Children's Centres, especially those frequented my women who otherwise lack access or the appropriate levels of digital literacies to connect to the kinds of existing, informal support available, might make available resources and advice for women to begin accessing online environments to find information, support and connect with others.

Such a strategy would also mean paying attention to the contextual factors surrounding the very many, varied, perinatal uses of technology, including difficulties in accessing these. This means paying particular attention to reaching out to specific needs of certain migrant mothers or mothers who may otherwise be excluded from even existing provisions. The ambition could also be to enable equipping healthcare professionals who do meet mothers offline, in their own homes or at Children's Centres, to develop a clear sense of the gaps being filled by existing digital provisions and of community and peer-led services already out there. This might then move towards a policy where resources can be recommended formally to mothers, when also alerting them to potential areas of caution, as discussed above in this book. In all potential versions of this, cross-sector cooperation between the NHS, communities, peer supporters and charities is critical.

A fundamentally crucial aspect of any digital strategy today is to recognise the changes that have accompanied the newest eras of the Web and the fact that with newer eras of digital spaces come a new set of opportunities and intrusions (Das & Ytre-Arne, 2018). A fuller engagement is key here, with newer eras of the Web, in responsible, engaged ways that stand for mothers' best interests and that move beyond envisaging websites as information sources alone, moving towards digital environments as active portals which can, with the many caveats as above, provide critical support in transitional twilight hours, both literally and metaphorically, in terms of their bridging roles, as discussed previously. Another suitable next step could perhaps be the designing of new, focused campaigns on perinatal well-being, including building on the NHS's repertoire of digital apps (see also Davies et al. 2017), for instance, and its history of interest in the role of social media technologies in women's health issues (see, for instance, Light & Ormandy, 2011). Designing these concrete, distinct digital campaigns, apps and services which fill gaps in provision, not by reinventing wheels but by beginning from where we are, through a concrete space for the maternal in a broader digital well-being strategy. This will come with its own needs for research and evaluation, of course, but it seems that a maternal digital well-being strategy in the context of NHS's digital strategy could make uses of existing, informal, online provisions, include new stand-alone environments and tools, combine offline and online provisions, exclude commercial encroachments entirely and address specific areas of perinatality, including but not restricted to conception and fertility, childbirth, infant feeding, infant sleep, family and relationship difficulties, financial difficulties, weaning, postnatal anxiety and postnatal depression. To end, the most critical and crucial point, of course, is money. Funding cuts do not help achieve any of this, but it does still help, I suggest, to place the digital and the perinatal on the list of priorities to consider for maternal well-being.

A (careful) case for the digital

In this final chapter, I have reflected upon findings from qualitative, face-to-face, online and offline research with women in the context of their everyday lives, trying to grasp the role of media technologies, particularly digital technologies, and environments in the context of perinatality. I have argued in the context of current research in digital health and well-being that digital perinatal or maternal well-being needs neither the reinvention of wheels nor great aspirations around the digital, but that balancing optimism and cautious perspectives might allow us to make a clear and strong case for the role of digital interfaces in filling critical, emerging gaps in perinatal support and well-being, at least in the U.K. I have argued here that recent austerity measures and funding cuts have resulted in evidenced gaps in provision which healthcare professionals, who are already focused on both mothers and infants or very young children (as opposed to mothers alone), are stretched, and provisions for mothers' emotional well-being but also wider forms of support around the myriad difficulties and challenges in the perinatal period are equally stretched. I have argued in this context that there is a need to balance optimism and caution when thinking about the promises and potentials of digital technologies in supporting mothers better in the perinatal period, and that digital 'solutions' need to blend seamlessly with better offline provision rather than being approached as a substitute.

Part of this balance, as I have suggested in this chapter, is to give maternal (not just perinatal) digital well-being a recognised and distinct space in an overall digital health and well-being strategy being pursued by the healthcare sector. While digital environments and interfaces developed around general health and well-being issues may be useful, the evidence that the early years brings specific social, physiological and emotional challenges for mothers and a frequent need for support and advice – more frequent and more 24/7 than can at the moment be provided through existing provisions – indicates that marrying the needs of the perinatal with aspirations around the digital could prove worthwhile. A balanced approach also means, as research within communication studies has consistently demonstrated, locating the online within and in relation to the offline. This means recognising inequalities of access, social and cultural factors standing in the way of engagement with online interfaces, differences in people's levels of literacies with these interfaces, particularly critical during the many moments of vulnerability in the perinatal period, and developing linkages between existing offline and online environments rather than solely beginning from scratch. A balanced approach also means remaining cautious, amidst the potentials of the digital in this context that not everyone will benefit equally and that social interaction in digital environments, like all mediated social interactions, can contribute to mixed levels of support and a range of emotional experiences.

This, of course, demands resources at all stages of the process, from conceptualisation through to evaluation, and it requires fundamentally more research and more resources and funding. Research is needed to understand more clearly the nature of needs in the perinatal period in a context-sensitive manner, including pronounced mental health needs, but also everyday needs around support for the very mundane but often isolating aspects of the very early years. Infant feeding, infant sleeping, weaning, baby weight gain are all issues which show up frequently on online discussion boards, where women, often themselves struggling to cope, support other women through difficult nights, for instance, at a time when telephone helplines (often very busy and difficult to reach) are inaccessible. More research is needed on what this chapter has called the gap-filling role of online support in the perinatal period, filling in the spaces between the need for support and physical face-to-face provision being able to meet that need, or in the periods where a new mother may find it difficult, socially, practically or even emotionally to go out to healthcare professionals and parent groups to socialize. More research is needed to locate these potential (and often arguable) benefits in the deeply contextualised, everyday contexts of mothers' lives, in order to deliver ambitions around culturally competent care, which means paying attention to inequalities of access as well as literacies. But, as this book has argued, there are critical gaps in provision for mothers at an evidenced, critical period in their lives, both in terms of maternal well-being and infant and wider family well-being. A balanced, context-sensitive and cautiously optimistic approach to researching existing, informal digital avenues of support and developing a space for maternal digital well-being in a digital strategic plan in the national health services in the U.K. would be a welcome and constructive step. Such a step must frame mothers as active agents and widely diverse in needs and practices, and any anticipated digital filling of gaps in provision must take into account not simply questions of access, but also literacies, online-offline linkages, inter-institutional cooperation, transparency, freedom from commercial encroachment and suitable mechanisms of evaluation. More importantly, it is imperative to be consciously distant from euphoric rhetoric around the potentials of the digital while making a case for and carving space for mothers, especially in the vulnerable periods of the perinatal in a digital strategy that is likely to continue to be significant.

Notes

1 I acknowledge here Louise Davies, Nadine Page and Victoria Redclift in alerting me to a few critical policy documents.

2 Accessed on 19 July 2019 on this link www.england.nhs.uk/mental-health/perinatal/community-services/

Bibliography

Abetz, J., & Moore, J. (2018). "Welcome to the mommy wars, ladies": Making sense of the ideology of combative mothering in mommy blogs. *Communication Culture & Critique, 11*(2), 265–281.

Adams, S. L. (2014). *Mad mothers, bad mothers, and what a "good" mother would do: The ethics of ambivalence.* New York: Columbia University Press.

Ahmed, S. (2004). Affective economies. *Social Text, 22*(2), 117–139.

Akass, K. (2012). Motherhood and Myth-Making: Despatches from the frontline of the US Mommy wars. *Feminist Media Studies, 12*(1), 137–141.

Almeida L. M., Costa-Santos C., Caldas J. P., Dias S., Ayres-de-Campos D. (2016). The impact of migration on women's mental health in the postpartum period. *Revista Saude Publica, 50*(35), 1–13. doi:10.1590/S1518-8787.2016050005617

Almond, P. & Lathlean, J. (2011), Inequity in provision of and access to health visiting postnatal depression services. *Journal of Advanced Nursing, 67*(11), 2350–2362.

Alper, M. (2019). Future talk: Accounting for the technological and other future discourses in daily life. *International Journal of Communication, 13*, 715–735.

Amichai-Hamburger, Y., & Furnham, A. (2007). The positive net. *Computers in Human Behavior, 23*(2), 1033–1045.

Amichai-Hamburger, Y., Kaynar, O. and Fine A. (2007). The effects of need for cognition on Internet use. *Computers in Human Behavior, 23*(1), 880–891.

Amichai-Hamburger, Y., Kingsbury, M., & Schneider, B. H. (2013). Friendship: An old concept with a new meaning?. *Computers in Human Behavior, 29*(1), 33–39.

Amichai-Hamburger, Y., Wainapel, G., & Fox, S. (2002). "On the internet no one knows I'm an introvert": Extroversion, neuroticism, and internet interaction. *Cyberpsychology & Behavior, 5*(2), 125–128.

Andersen, B., & Parker-Ward, S. (2019). From awareness to advocacy: A two-year analysis of prenatal and maternal health conversations on social media. Paper presented at the International Communication Association Conference, Washington, DC, May 2019.

Andreassen, R. (2017). New kinships, new family formations and negotiations of intimacy via social media sites. *Journal of Gender Studies, 26*(3), 1–11.

Andreassen, R., Raun, T., Harrison, K., & Petersen, M. N. (2017). Introduction: Mediated intimacies. In R. Andreassen, M. N. Petersen, K. Harrison & T. Raun (eds.) *Mediated intimacies* (pp. 1–16). London: Routledge.

AOIR (2012). Ethical decision-making and internet research. https://aoir.org/reports/ethics2.pdf

Asher, R. (2011). *Shattered: modern motherhood and the illusion of equality.* London: Harvill Secker.

Arendell, T. (2000). Conceiving and investigating motherhood: The decade's scholarship. *Journal of Marriage and Family, 62*(4), 1192–1207.

Arendt, H. (1958). *The human condition.* Chicago, IL: University of Chicago Press.

Babatunde, T. & Moreno-Leguizamon, C. J. (2012). Daily and cultural issues of postnatal depression in African women immigrants in South-East London: Tips for health professionals. *Nursing Research and Practice*, doi:10.1155/2012/181640.

Badinter, E. (2012). *The conflict: How modern motherhood undermines the status of women.* New York: Palgrave Macmillan.

Bakardjieva, M. (2005). *Internet society: The internet in everyday life.* London: Sage.

Bamberg, S. Hunecke, M., & Blobaum, A. (2007). Social context, personal norms and the use of public transportation: Two field studies. *Journal of Environmental Psychology, 27*(3), 190–203.

Bang, R. A., Bang, A. T., Reddy, M. H., Deshmukh, M. D., Baitule, S. B., & Filippi, V. (2004). Maternal morbidity during labour and the puerperium in rural homes and the need for medical attention: a prospective observational study in Gadchiroli, India. *BJOG: An International Journal of Obstetrics & Gynaecology, 111*(3), 231–238.

Baraitser, L. (2009). Mothers who make things public. *Feminist review, 93*(1), 8–26.

Baraitser, L. (2017). YouTube birth and the primal scene. *Performance Research, 22*(4), 7–17.

Barak, A., & Gluck-Ofri, O. (2007). Degree and reciprocity of self-disclosure in online forums. *CyberPsychology & Behavior, 10*(3), 407–417.

Barassi, V. (2017). BabyVeillance? Expecting parents, online surveillance and the cultural specificity of pregnancy apps. *Social Media + Society, 3*(2), doi: 10.1177/2056305117707188.

Barnes, C., & Power, M. (2015). Internalising discourses of parenting blame: Voices from the field. *Studies in the Maternal, 4*(2), 1–21.

Baumann, E., Czerwinski, F., & Reifegerste, D. (2017). Gender-specific determinants and patterns of online health information seeking: Results from a representative German health survey. *Journal of Medical Internet Research, 19*(4), e92.

Baym, N. K. (2015). *Personal connections in the digital age.* Cambridge, UK: Polity Press.

BBC. (2016). Huge gaps in mental health care for new mothers. Retrieved from www.bbc.co.uk/news/health-28182375 on 12.04.2017.

BBC. (2018). Perinatal mental health: No specialist unit 'detrimental' to new mums. https://www.bbc.co.uk/news/av/uk-wales-44585962/perinatal-mental-health-no-specialist-unit-detrimental-to-new-mums

Beck, U. (1992). Risk society: *Towards a new modernity.* London: Sage.

Beck, U., & Beck-Gernsheim, E. (2001). *Individualization.* London: Sage.

Beck, U., Giddens, A., & Lash, S. (1994). *Reflexive modernization.* Stanford: Stanford University Press.

Bernhardt, J. M., & Felter, E. M. (2004). Online pediatric information seeking among mothers of young children: Results from a qualitative study using focus groups. *Journal of Medical Internet Research, 6*(1), e7.

Betterton, R. (2009). Maternal bodies in visual culture. *Studies in the Maternal, 1*(1), 1–3.

Bion, W. R. (1965). *Transformations.* London: Karnac.

Bird, E. S. (2003). *The audience of everyday life.* New York & London: Routledge.

Blum-Ross, A., & Livingstone, S. (2017). "Sharenting," parent blogging, and the boundaries of the digital self. *Popular Communication, 15*(2), 110–125.

Bochantin, J. E., Broadfoot, K. J., Bute, J. J., Buzzanell, P., Cowan, R. L., Cunningham, S. R., & Fixmer-Oraiz, N. (2010). *Contemplating maternity in an era of choice: Explorations into discourses of reproduction.* Lanham, MD: Lexington Books.

Bohn, K. (2017). Babies of anxious moms focus more on threats. *Futurity.org.* Retrieved from www.futurity.org/babies-anxious-moms-threats-1556992/ on 2 August 2018.

Bourdieu, P. (1985). The social space and the genesis of groups. *Information (International Social Science Council), 24*(2), 195–220.

Brady, E., & Guerin, S. (2010). "Not the romantic, all happy, coochy coo experience": Aqualitative analysis of interactions on an Irish parenting web site. *Family Relations, 59*(1), 14–27.

British Medical Association. (2018). *Lost in transit? Funding for mental health services in England.* London: BMA.

Brodie, M., Flournoy, R. E., Altman, D. E., Blendon, R. J., Benson, J. M., & Rosenbaum, M. D. (2000). Health information, the Internet, and the Digital Divide. *Health Affairs, 19*, 255–265.

Brooks, R., & Hodkinson, P. (2019). Out-of-place: The lack of engagement with parent networks of caregiving fathers of young children. *Families, Relationships and Societies.*

Brown, W. (2015). *Undoing the demos: Neoliberalism's stealth revolution.* New York: Zone Books.

Brubaker, S. J., & Dillaway, H. E. (2009). Medicalization, natural childbirth and birthing experiences. *Sociology Compass, 3*(1), 31–48.

Bruer, J. T. (1999). *The myth of the first three years.* New York: The Free Press.

Brunet, P. M., & Schmidt, L. A. (2007). Is shyness context specific? Relation between shyness and online self-disclosure with and without a live webcam in young adults. *Journal of Research in Personality, 41*(4), 938–945.

Bucher, T. (2017). The algorithmic imaginary: Exploring the ordinary affects of Facebook algorithms. *Information, Communication & Society, 20*(1), 30–44.

Burgess, J., & Green, J. (2013). *YouTube: Online video and participatory culture.* Chichester: John Wiley & Sons.

Bute, J. J. (2009). "Nobody thinks twice about asking": Women with a fertility problem and requests for information. *Health communication, 24*(8), 752–763.

Bute, J. J., Vik, T. A. (2010). Privacy management as unfinished business: Shifting boundaries in the context of infertility. *Communication Studies, 61*(1), 1–20.

Butler, J. (1997). *Excitable speech: A politics of the performative.* New York: Psychology Press.

Butler, K. (2010). Intensive mothering in British Columbia: Understanding the impact of an "investing-in-children" framework on mothering ideology. *International Journal of Canadian Studies, 42*, 243–253.

Caplan, S. E., & Turner, J. S. (2007). Bringing theory to research on computer-mediated comforting communication. *Computers in Human Behavior, 23*(2), 985–998.

Cappellini, B., & Yen, D. A. W. (2016). A space of one's own: Spatial and identity liminality in an online community of mothers. *Journal of Marketing Management, 32*(13–14), 1260–1283.

Carlisle, S. & Hanlon, P. (2008). Well-being and consumer culture: A different kind of public problem? *Health Promotion International.*

Carlisle, C., Calman, L., & Ibbotson, T. (2009). Practice-based learning: the role of practice education facilitators in supporting mentors. *Nurse Education Today.*

Chadwick, R. J., & Foster, D. (2013). Technologies of gender and childbirth choices: Home birth, elective caesarean and white femininities in South Africa. *Feminism & Psychology, 23*(3), 317–338.

Chae, J. (2015). "Am I a better mother than you?". *Communication Research, 42*(4), 503–525.

Chalklen, C., & Anderson, H. (2017). Mothering on Facebook: Exploring the privacy/openness paradox. *Social Media+ Society, 3*(2), doi:10.1177/2056305117707187

Chambers, D. (2013). *Social media and personal relationships: Online intimacies and networked friendship.* New York, NY: Springer.

Chambers, D. (2016). Networked intimacy: Algorithmic friendship and scalable sociality. *European Journal of Communication*, 32, 26–36.

Chan, A. H. (2008). 'Life in happy land': Using virtual space and doing motherhood in Hong Kong. *Gender, Place & Culture, 15*(2), 169–188. doi:10.1080/09663690701863281

Chen, G. M. (2013). Don't call me that: A techno-feminist critique of the term mommy blogger. *Mass Communication and Society, 16*(4), 510–532. doi:10.1080/15205436.2012.737888

Chen, G. M. (2015). Why do women bloggers use social media? Recreation and information motivations outweigh engagement motivations. *New Media & Society, 17*(1), 24–40. doi:10.1177/1461444813504269

Cheresheva, I. (2015). Food for thought: A comparative analysis of online narratives of maternal practices of infant feeding in Hungary and Bulgaria. *Women's Studies International Forum, 53*, 147–158. http://ezproxy3.lib.le.ac.uk/; doi:10.1016/j.wsif.2014.10.022

Choe, E. K., Lee, N. B., Lee, B., Pratt, W., & Kientz, J. A. (2014). Understanding quantified selfers' practices in collecting and exploring personal data. In *Proceedings of the Thirty Second Annual ACM Conference on Human Factors in Computing Systems*, Toronto, Canada, 26 April–1 May, 2014, pp. 1143–1152.

Cline, R. J. W., & Haynes, K. M. (2001). Consumer health information seeking on the internet: The state of the art. *Health Education Research, 16*, 671–692. doi:10.1093/her/16.6.671

Coffey, A., Beverley, H., & Paul, A. (1996). Qualitative data analysis: Technologies and representations. *Sociological Research Online, 1*(1), 1–12.

Coleman, J. S. (1988). Social capital in the creation of human capital. *American Journal of Sociology, 94*, S95–S120.

Coltrane, S. (2010). Gender theory and household labor. *Sex Roles*, 63, 791–800.

Cooley, C. H. (1902). Looking-glass self. In J. O'Brien (ed.) *The production of reality: Chapters and readings on social interaction* (p. 6). Thousand Oaks, CA: Pine Forge Press.

Coontz, S. (1997). *The way we really are: Coming to terms with America's changing family.* New York: Basic Books.

Couldry, N. (2004). Theorising media as practice. *Social Semiotics, 14*(2), 114–132.

Couldry, N. (2008). Mediatization or mediation? Alternative understandings of the emergent space of digital storytelling. *New Media & Society, 10*(3), 373–391.

Couldry, N., & Hepp, A. (2016). *The mediated construction of reality*. Cambridge, UK: Polity Press.

Couldry, N., & Hepp, A. (2018). The continuing lure of the mediated centre in times of deep mediatization: Media events and its enduring legacy. *Media, Culture & Society, 40*(1), 114–117.

Cripe, E. T. (2017). "You can't bring your cat to work": Challenges mothers face combining breastfeeding and working. *Qualitative Research Reports in Communication, 18*(1), 36–44.

Dahlen, H. G., & Homer, C. S. E. (2013). "Motherbirth or childbirth"? A prospective analysis of vaginal birth after caesarean blogs. *Midwifery, 29*(2), 167. doi:10.1016/j.midw.2011.11.007

Dalmiya, V., & Alcoff, L. (1993). Are "old wives' tales" justified?. *Feminist Epistemologies, 1993*, 217–244.

Das, R. (2017a). The mediation of childbirth: "Joyful" birthing and strategies of silencing on a Facebook discussion group. *European Journal of Cultural Studies*. doi:10.1177/1367549417722094.

Das, R. (2017b). Speaking about birth: Visible and silenced narratives in online discussions of childbirth. *Social Media+ Society, 3*(4). doi:10.1177/2056305117735753.

Das, R. (2018a). *The internet and maternal wellbeing*. London: Routledge.

Das, R. (2018b). Mediated subjectivities of the maternal: A critique of childbirth videos on YouTube. *The Communication Review, 21*(1), 66–84.

Das, R. (2018c). *The mediation of childbirth: Birth Stories*. London: Routledge.

Das, R. (2018d). Temporally inexpensive, affectively expensive: Digitally-mediated maternal interpersonal ties in the perinatal months. *Communication Culture & Critique, 11*(4), 586–603.

Das, R. (2019). Mothers' day: Ambivalences, uncertainties and fractures of mother. Surrey Sociology Blog.http://blogs.surrey.ac.uk/sociology/2019/03/28/mothers-day-ambivalences-fractures-and-ambiguities-of-mother/

Das, R. & Hodkinson, P. (2019). Tapestries of intimacy: Networked intimacies and new fathers' emotional self-disclosure of mental health struggles. *Social Media and Society*. doi: 10.1177/2056305119846488.

Das, R., & Ytre-Arne, B. (2018). An agenda in the interest of audiences: Facing the challenges of intrusive media technologies. *Television and New Media*. 20(2), doi: 10.1177/1527476418759604.

Davidson, J., & Milligan, C. (2004). Embodying emotion sensing space: Introducing emotional geographies. *Social & Cultural Geography, 5*(4), 523–532.

Davies, E. B., Craven, M. P., Martin, J. L., & Simons, L. (2017). Proportionate methods for evaluating a simple digital mental health tool. *Evidence-Based Mental Health, 20*(4), 112–117.

De Benedictis, S. (2012). Feral parents: Austerity parenting under neoliberalism. *Studies in the Maternal, 4*(2), 1–21.

De Benedictis, S. (2017). Watching one born every minute: Negotiating the terms of the "good birth". In R. Mosely, H. Wheatley & H. Wood (eds.) *Television for women: New directions* (pp. 110–127). Abingdon/New York: Routledge.

Deyl, S. (2017). Maneka Gandhi calls caesarean section surgeries a racket. *The Times News Network*. Retrieved from http://timesofindia.indiatimes.com/india/alarming-rise-in-caesarean-sections/chaptershow/57302940.cms on 24.07.2017.

DoH (Department of Health). (2011). *Health visitor implementation plan 2011–2015*. London: Department of Health.

Douglas, S., & Michaels, M. (2005). *The mommy myth: The idealization of motherhood and how it has undermined all women.* New York: Simon & Schuster.

Downing, G. (2008). A different way to help. *Human development in the twenty-first century* (pp. 200–205). Cambridge: Cambridge University Press.

Drentea, P. & Moren-Cross, J. L. (2005). Social capital and social support on the web: The case of an internet mother site. *Sociology of Health & Illness, 27*(7), 920–943.

Du Gay, P. (1997). *Production of culture/cultures of production.* London: Sage.

Duffy, B. (2015). Amateur, autonomous, and collaborative: Myths of aspiring female cultural producers in Web 2.0. *Critical Studies in Media Communication, 32*(1), 48–64.

Edge, D. (2007a). Ethnicity, psychosocial risk, and perinatal depression – A comparative study among inner-city women in the United Kingdom. *Journal of Psychosomatic Research, 63*, 291–295.

Edge, D. (2007b). Perinatal depression and Black Caribbean women: Lessons for primary care. *Primary Health Care, 17*, 32–35.

Edge, D. (2010). Falling through the net – Black and minority ethnic women and perinatal mental healthcare: Health professionals' views. *General Hospital Psychiatry, 32*(1), 17–25.

Edge, D. (2011). *National perinatal mental health project report.* London: National Mental Health Development Unit.

Edwards, R. (2004). Present and absent in troubling ways: Families and social capital debates. *The Sociological Review, 52*(1), 1–21.

Elliott, H. (2011). Interviewing mothers: Reflections on closeness and reflexivity in research encounters. *Studies in the Maternal, 3*(1), 94–122.

Elliott, S., Powell, R., & Brenton, J. (2015). Being a good mom. *Journal of Family Issues, 36*(3), 351–370. doi:10.1177/0192513X13490279

Ellison, N. B., Steinfield, C., & Lampe, C. (2007). The benefits of Facebook "friends:" Social capital and college students' use of online social network sites. *Journal of Computer-Mediated Communication, 12*(4), 1143–1168.

Ellison, N. B., Steinfeld, C., & Lampe, C. (2008). Social capital, self-esteem, and use of online social network sites. *Journal of Applied Developmental Psychology, 29*(6), 434–445.

Escobar, A. (1994). Welcome to Cyberia: Notes on the anthropology of cyberculture. *Current Anthropology, 35*, 211–232.

Fage-Butler, A. M. (2017). Risk resistance: Constructing home birth as morally responsible on an online discussion group. *Health, Risk & Society, 19*(3–4), 130–144.

Faircloth, C. (2010). "If they want to risk the health and well-being of their child, that's up to them": Long-term breastfeeding, risk and maternal identity. *Health, Risk & Society, 12*(4), 357–367.

Faircloth, C. (2013). 'Intensive motherhood' in Comparative perspective: Feminism, full-term breastfeeding and attachment parenting in London and Paris (Chapter 7). In C. Faircloth, Diane M. Hoffman & Linda L. Layne (eds.) *Parenting in global perspective: Negotiating ideologies of kinship, self and politics.* Relationships and resources. London: Routledge.

Faircloth, C. (2013). *Militant lactivism?: Attachment parenting and intensive motherhood in the UK and France* (Vol. 24). Oxford: Berghahn Books.

Faircloth, C. (2017). "Natural" breastfeeding in comparative perspective: Feminism, morality, and adaptive accountability. *Ethnos, 82*(1), 19–43.

Faircloth, C., & Gürtin, Z. B. (2018). Fertile connections: Thinking across assisted reproductive technologies and parenting culture studies. *Sociology*, *52*(5), 983–1000.

Feldman, R., Granat, A., Pariente, C., Kanety, H., Kuint, J., & Gilboa-Schechtman, E. (2009). Maternal depression and anxiety across the postpartum year and infant social engagement, fear regulation, and stress reactivity. *Journal of the American Academy of Child & Adolescent Psychiatry, 48*(9), 919–927.

Fox, B. (2009). *When Couples Become Parents: The Creation of Gender in the Transition to Parenthood.* Toronto: University of Toronto Press.

Friedlander, L. (2008). Narrative strategies in a digital age: Authorship and authority. In *Digital Storytelling, Mediatized Stories: Self-Representations in New Media* (pp. 177–194). New York: Peter Lang Publishing, Inc.

Fuchs, C., Hofkirchner, W., Schafranek, M., Raffl, C., Sandoval, M., & Bichler, R. (2010). Theoretical foundations of the web: Cognition, communication and co-operation. Towards an Understanding of the Web. *Future Internet*, *2*(1), 41–59.

Furedi, F. (2001). *Paranoid Parenting.* London: Penguin.

Furedi, F. (2006a). Cotton wool kids? Making sense of "child safety". *Generation Youth Issues*, *4*, 4–6.

Furedi, F. (2006b). *Culture of fear revisited.* New York: A&C Black.

Furedi, F. (2008). Fear and security: A vulnerability-led policy response. *Social Policy and Administration*, *42*(6), 645–661.

Gadamer, H. G. (2002). *The beginning of knowledge.* New York, NY: Bloomsbury Publishing.

Gajjala, R. (2015). When your seams get undone, do you learn to sew or to kill monsters?. *The Communication Review, 18*(1), 23–36.

Gaskin, I. M. (2003). Going backwards: The concept of "pasmo". *The Practising Midwife, 6*(8), 34–37.

Gedalof, I. (2009). Birth, belonging and migrant mothers: Narratives of reproduction in feminist migration studies. *Feminist Review, 93*(1), 81–100.

Georgakopoulou, A. (2007). *Small Stories, Interaction and Identities.* Amsterdam; Philadelphia, PA: John Benjamins Pub. Co.

Giddens, A. (1991a). *The Consequences of Modernity.* Cambridge, UK: Polity Press.

Giddens, A. (1991b). *Modernity and self-identity: Self and society in the late modern age.* Stanford, CA: Stanford University Press.

Giddens, A. (2013). *The transformation of intimacy: Sexuality, love and eroticism in modern societies.* Oxford: John Wiley & Sons.

Gill, R. (2007). Postfeminist media culture: Elements of a sensibility. *European Journal of Cultural Studies, 10*(2), 147–166.

Gill, R., & Orgad, S. (2016). The confidence cult(ure). *Australian Feminist Studies, 30*(86), 324–344.

Gillies, V. (2007). *Marginalised mothers: Exploring working class experiences.* London: Routledge.

Giroux, H. A. (2008). *Against the terror of neoliberalism: Politics beyond the age of greed.* London: Routledge.

Gong, G. (2016). *Children's healthcare and parental media engagement in urban China: A culture of anxiety.* Basingstoke: Palgrave Macmillan.

Gonzalez-Polledo, E., & Tarr, J. (2016). The thing about pain: The remaking of illness narratives in chronic pain expressions on social media. *New Media & Society, 18*(8), 1455–1472. doi:10.1177/1461444814560126

Granovetter, M. S. (1973). The strength of weak ties. *American Journal of Sociology, 78*(6), 1360–1380.

Gray, J. (2013). Feeding on the web: Online social support in the breastfeeding context. *Communication Research Reports, 30*(1), 1–11. doi:10.1080/08824096.2012.746219

Greenhalgh, T. & Keen, J. (2014). *"Personalising" NHS information technology in England.* Editorial: BMJ.

Greenhalgh, T., Procter, R., Wherton, J., Sugarhood, P., & Shaw, S. (2012). The organising vision for telehealth and telecare: Discourse analysis. *BMJ Open, 2*(4). doi:10.1136/bmjopen-2012-001574

Hamilton, P. (2017) *"We do this too": Black mothers' engagements with attachment parenting in Britain and Canada.* Unpublished thesis. University of Western Ontario.

Hanser, A., & Li, J. (2017). The hard work of feeding the baby: Breastfeeding and intensive mothering in contemporary urban China. *The Journal of Chinese Sociology, 4*(1), 4–18.

Hanson, C. (2004). *A Cultural History of Pregnancy: Pregnancy, Medicine and Culture, 1750–2000.* Berlin: Springer.

Hardey, M. (2010). Digital medicine: Health care in the internet era. *Sociology of Health and Illness, 32*(2), 506–507.

Harman, V., & Cappellini, B. (2015). Mothers on display: Lunchboxes, social class and moral accountability. *Sociology, 49*(4), 764–781.

Harman, V., Cappellini, B., & Faircloth, C. (2019). *Feeding children inside and outside the home: Critical perspectives* (216 pp.). London: British Sociological Association; Routledge.

Harmsen, I. A., Doorman, G. G., Mollema, L., Ruiter, R. A. C., Kok, G., & de Melker, H. E. (2013). Parental information – Seeking behaviour in childhood vaccinations. BMC Public Health, 13, 1219. doi:10.1186/1471-2458-13-1219

Harris, J. R. (1998). *The nurture assumption.* New York: The Free Press.

Harvey, J. (2016). Implementing scalable digital healthcare solutions in England: Is the condition of society a factor? *Information, Communication & Society, 19*(4), 532–539.

Hausman, B. (2005). Risky business: Framing childbirth in hospital settings. *Journal of Medical Humanities, 26*(1), 23–38.

Hawn, C. (2009). Take two aspirin and tweet me in the morning: How twitter, Facebook, and other social media are reshaping health care. *Health Affairs (Project Hope), 28*(2), 361. doi:10.1377/hlthaff.28.2.361

Hays, S. (1996). *The Cultural Contradictions of Motherhood.* New Haven & London: Yale University Press.

Hays, S. (1998). *The Cultural Contradictions of Motherhood.* New Haven, CT: Yale University Press.

Haythornthwaite, C. (2002). Strong, weak, and latent ties and the impact of new media. *The Information Society, 18*(5), 385–401.

Haythornthwaite, C. A., & Wellman, B. (Eds.). (2002). *The Internet in Everyday Life* (pp. 3–42). Oxford: Blackwell.

Helfer, R. E. (1987). The perinatal period, a window of opportunity for enhancing parent-infant communication: An approach to prevention. *Child Abuse & Neglect, 11*(4), 565–579.

Henderson, A., Harmon, S., & Newman, H. (2016). The price mothers pay, even when they are not buying it: Mental health consequences of idealized motherhood. *Sex Roles, 74*(11–12), 512–526.

Henwood, K., Pidgeon, N., Sarre, S., Simmons, P., & Smith, N. (2008). Risk, framing and everyday life: Epistemological and methodological reflections from three socio-cultural projects. *Health, Risk & Society, 10*(5), 421–438.

Hern, A. 2019. Parenting club Bounty fined £400,000 for selling users' data. *The Guardian.* www.theguardian.com/technology/2019/apr/12/parenting-club-bounty-fined-selling-users-data (link last accessed on 16/07/2019)

Hether, H. J., Murphy, S. T., & Valente, T. W. (2014). It's better to give than to receive: The role of social support, trust, and participation on health-related social networking sites. *Journal of Health Communication, 19*(12), 1424–1439. doi:10.1080/10810730.2014.894596

Hewitt, P. L., & Flett, G. L. (1991). Perfectionism in the self and social contexts: Conception, assessment, and the association with psychopathology. *Journal of Personality and Social Psychology, 60*, 456–470.

Hills, P. & Argyle, M. (2003). Uses of the internet and their relationships with individual differences in personality. *Computers in Human Behavior, 19*(1), 59–70.

Hobbs, R. (1998). The seven great debates in the media literacy movement. *Journal of Communication, 48*(1), 16–32.

Hodkinson, P., & Brooks, R. (2018). Interchangeable parents?. The roles and identities of primary and equal carer fathers of young children. *Current Sociology.* doi:10.1177/0011392118807530

Hogan, B. (2010). The presentation of self in the age of social media: Distinguishing performances and exhibitions online. *Bulletin of Science, Technology & Society, 30*(6), 377–386.

Hogan, S., & Pink, S. (2012). Visualising interior worlds. In S. Pink (ed.) *Advances in Visual Methodology* (230–247). London: Sage.

Hollway, W. (2001). From motherhood to maternal subjectivity. *International Journal of Critical Psychology, 2*, 13–38.

Hope, J. (2015). Anxiety is catching. *The Mail Online.* Retrieved from www.dailymail.co.uk/health/chapter-3053778/Anxiety-catching-passed-children-scientists-warn-protective-parents.html on 02.08.2018.

Horeck, T. (2016). The affective labour of one born every minute in its UK and US formats. *Critical Studies in Television, 11*(2), 164–176.

Hsiao, J. C. Y., & Dillahunt, T. R. (2017, February). People-nearby applications: How newcomers move their relationships offline and develop social and cultural capital. 20th ACM Conference on Computer-Supported Cooperative Work (pp. 26–40).

Hunt, D., Koteyko, N., & Gunter, B. (2015). UK policy on social networking sites and online health: From informed patient to informed consumer?. *Digital Health*, 1. doi:10.1177/2055207615592513

Hunter, A. (2016). Monetizing the mommy: Mommy blogs and the audience commodity. *Information, Communication & Society, 19*(9), 1306–1320. doi:10.1080/1369118X.2016.1187642

Independent Mental Health Taskforce. (2016). *The five year forward view for mental health predict.* Leeds: NHS England.

Jacobs, A. (2007). *On matricide: Myth, psychoanalysis and the law of the mother.* New York: Columbia University Press.

Jarrett, K. (2014). The relevance of "women's work" social reproduction and immaterial labor in digital media. *Television & New Media, 15*(1), 14–29.

Jensen, T. (2012). Tough Love in Tough Times. *Studies in the Maternal*, 4(2), 1–26.

Jensen, T. (2013). "Mumsnetiquette": Online affect within parenting culture. In C. Maxwell & P. Aggleton (eds.) *Privilege, agency and affect* (pp. 127–145). London: Palgrave Macmillan.

Jensen, T., & Tyler, I. (2012). Austerity parenting: New economies of parent-citizenship. *Studies in the Maternal*, *4*(2), 1–5.

Johnson, S. A. (2015). "Intimate mothering publics": Comparing face-to-face support groups and internet use for women seeking information and advice in the transition to first-time motherhood. *Culture, Health & Sexuality, 17*(2), 237–251. doi:10.1080/13691058.2014.968807

Jones, S. (Ed.). (1998). *Doing internet research: Critical issues and methods for examining the net.* London: Sage.

Katz, J. E., & Rice, R. E. (2002). *Social consequences of internet use: Access, involvement, and interaction.* Cambridge, MA: MIT Press.

Keenan, J., & Stapleton, H. (2010). Bonny babies? Motherhood and nurturing in the age of obesity. *Health, Risk & Society, 12*(4), 369–383.

Kim, J., & Lee, S. (2014). Communication and cybercoping: Coping with chronic illness through communicative action in online support networks. *Journal of Health Communication, 19*(7), 775–794. doi:10.1080/10810730.2013.864724

Kitzinger, S. (2012a). *The new experience of childbirth.* London: Hachette.

Kitzinger, S. (2012b). Rediscovering the social model of childbirth. *Birth, 39*(4), 301–304.

Klassen, P. E. (2001). *Blessed events: Religion and home birth in America.* Princeton, NJ: Princeton University Press.

Kleut, J. Picone, I, Pavlickova, T. Bojana, R. Moller Hartley, J., & De Ridder, S. (2018). Small acts of engagement: Reconnecting productive audience practices with everyday agency. *New Media and Society, 21*(9), doi: 10.1177/1461444819837569.

Klinnert. M.D. & Robinson, J.L. (2008). Addressing the psychological needs of families of food-allergic children. *Current Allergy and Asthma Reports, 8*(3), 196–200.

Koteyko, N., Hunt, D., & Gunter, B. (2015). Expectations in the field of the internet and health: An analysis of claims about social networking sites in clinical literature. *Sociology of Health & Illness, 37*(3), 468–484.

Kress, G. R. (2003). *Literacy in the new media age.* New York: Psychology Press.

Kristeva, J. (1989). *Black Sun: Depression and Melancholia.* New York: Columbia University Press.

Kristeva, J., & Goldhammer, A. (1985). Stabat mater. *Poetics Today, 6*, 133–152.

Lambert, J. (2006). *Digital storytelling cookbook: February 2007.* Berkeley, CA: Digital Diner Press.

Larner, W. (2000). Neo-liberalism: Policy, ideology, governmentality. *Studies in Political Economy. 63*, 5–25.

Latif, Z. (2014). The maternal mental health of migrant women. A race equality foundation briefing chapter. *Better Health Briefing 31.*

Lawler, S. (2002). Narratives in social research. In T. May (ed.) *Qualitative research in action* (pp. 242–258). London: Sage.

Leahy-Warren, P., McCarthy, G., & Corcoran, P. (2011). Postnatal depression in first-time mothers: Prevalence and relationships between functional and structural social support at 6 and 12 weeks postpartum. *Archives of Psychiatric Nursing, 25*(3), 174–184.

Leaver, T. (2015). Born digital? Presence, privacy, and intimate surveillance. In J. Hartley & W. Qu (eds.) *Re-orientation: Translingual transcultural transmedia. Studies in narrative, language, identity, and knowledge* (pp. 149–160). Shanghai: Fudan University Press.

Leaver, T. & Highfield, T. (2016). Instagrammatics and digital methods. *Communication Research and Practice*, (2), 47–62.

Leavitt, J. W. (1986). Under the shadow of maternity: American women's responses to death and debility fears in nineteenth-century childbirth. *Feminist Studies, 12*(1), 129–154.

Lee, E. J. (2008). Living with risk in the age of "intensive motherhood": Maternal identity and infant feeding. *Health, Risk & Society, 10*(5), 467–477. doi:10.1080/13698570802383432

Lee, E. J., Bristow J., Faircloth C., & MacVarish J. (2014). *Parenting Culture Studies.* Basingstoke: Macmillan.

Lehman, S. (2014). Babies of anxious mothers are more likely to cry excessively. *Reuters.* Retrieved from www.reuters.com/chapter/us-maternal-anxiety-crying/babies-of-anxious-mothers-more-likely-to-cry-excessively-study-idUSKBN0FQ-1ZW20140721 on 02.08.2018

Ley, B. L. (2007). Vive les roses!: The architecture of commitment in an online pregnancy and mothering group. *Journal of Computer-Mediated Communication, 12*(4), 1388–1408.

Light, B., & Ormandy, P. (2011). *Lesbian, gay and bisexual women in the north-west: A multi-method study of cervical screening attitudes, experiences and uptake.* Salford: University of Salford.

Litt, J. S. (2000). *Medicalized motherhood: Perspectives from the lives of African-American and Jewish women.* New Brunswick: Rutgers University Press.

Lister, M. and Wells, L. (2008). *Seeing beyond belief.* Eng 242.

Littler, J. (2013). The rise of the "yummy mummy": Popular conservatism and the neoliberal maternal in contemporary British culture. *Communication, Culture & Critique*, 6(2), 227–243.

Littler, J. (2019). Mothers behaving badly: Chaotic hedonism and the crisis of neoliberal social reproduction. *Cultural Studies*, 1–22.

Livingstone, S. (2004). Media literacy and the challenge of new information and communication technologies. *The Communication Review*, 7(1), 3–14.

Livingstone, S. (2008). On the mediation of everything: ICA presidential address 2008. *Journal of Communication, 59*(1), 1–18.

Livingstone, S. (2009). *Children and the internet.* Cambridge, UK: Polity Press.

Livingstone, S. (2013). The participation paradigm in audience research. *Communication Review, 16*, 1–2, 21–30.

Locatelli, E. (2017). Images of breastfeeding on instagram: Self-representation, publicness, and privacy management. *Social Media and Society, 3*(2).

Longhurst, R. (2009a). *Maternities: Genders, bodies and space.* London: Routledge.

Longhurst, R. (2009b). YouTube: A new space for birth?. *Feminist Review, 93*(1), 46–63.

Lopez, L. K. (2009). The radical act of "mommy blogging": Redefining motherhood through the blogosphere. *New Media & Society, 11*(5), 729–747. doi:10.1177/1461444809105349

Luce, A., Cash, M., Hundley, V., Cheyne, H., Van Teijlingen, E., & Angell, C. (2016). "Is it realistic?" the portrayal of pregnancy and childbirth in the media. *BMC Pregnancy and Childbirth, 16*(1), Article no. 40. https://bmcpregnancychildbirth.biomedcentral.com/articles/10.1186/s12884-016-0827-x.

Lundby, K. (2008). *Digital Storytelling, Mediatized Stories: Self-representations in New Media* (Vol. 52). New York: Peter Lang.

Lupton, D. (1998). *The emotional self.* London: Sage.

Lupton, D. (1999). Risk and the ontology of pregnant embodiment. In: D. Lupton (ed.) *Risk and Sociocultural Theory: New Directions and Perspectives* (pp. 59–85). Cambridge, UK: Cambridge University Press.

Lupton, D. (2018). *Digital health: Critical and cross-disciplinary perspectives.* London: Routledge.

Lupton, D. (2012a). Beyond the "affect heuristic": The emotion-risk assemblage. Retrieved from https://ses.library.usyd.edu.au/bitstream/handle/2123/8794/TASA%20-%20Risk%20and%20Emotion.pdf;jsessionid=D8B8B1E904E9AB0E056DA96723E2BF9E?sequence=2

Lupton, D. (2012b). "Precious cargo": Foetal subjects, risk and reproductive citizenship. *Critical Public Health*, 22(3), 329–340.

Lupton, D. (2014). Apps as artefacts: Towards a critical perspective on mobile health and medical apps. *Societies, 4*(4), 606–622.

Lupton, D. (2016). "Mastering your fertility" – The digitised reproductive citizen. Forthcoming in A. McCosker, S. Vivienne & A. Johns (eds.) *Negotiating Digital Citizenship: Control, Contest and Culture* (pp. 81–93). London: Rowman and Littlefield. Preprint version available at: https://chapters.ssrn.com/sol3/chapters.cfm?abstract_id=2679402

Lupton, D. (2017). Feeling data: Touch and data sense. *Forthcoming in New Media & Society.* Retrieved from https://simplysociology.files.wordpress.com/2017/03/lupton-2017-feeling-data-touch-anddata-sense.pdf

Lupton, D., Pedersen, S., & Thomas, G. (2016). Parenting and digital media: From the early web to contemporary digital society. *Sociology Compass, 10*(8), 730–743.

Lwe, E. J. (2008). Living with risk in the age of "intensive motherhood": Maternal identity and infant feeding. *Health, Risk & Society, 10*(5), 467–477.

Mack, A. N. (2016). The self-made mom: Neoliberalism and masochistic motherhood in home-birth videos on YouTube. *Women's Studies in Communication, 39*(1), 47–68.

MacKenzie, D., & Wajcman, J. (1999). *The social shaping of technology.* Buckingham: Open University Press.

Macvarish, J. (2010). The effect of 'risk-thinking' on the contemporary construction of teenage motherhood. *Health, Risk & Society, 12*(4), 313–322.

Macvarish, J., & Lee, E. J. (2019). Constructions of parents in adverse childhood experiences discourse. *Social Policy and Society, 18*(3), 467–477. ISSN 1474-7464; doi:10.1017/S1474746419000083

Macvarish, J., Lee, E., & Sheldon, S. (2013). The role of counsellors in infertility clinics. *BioNews.* http://www.bionews.org.uk/page_249841.asp?

Madge, C., & O'Connor, H. (2006). Parenting gone wired: Empowerment of new mothers on the internet?. *Social and Cultural Geography*, 7(2), 199–220. http://hdl.handle.net/2381/1403; doi:10.1080/14649360600600528

Madianou, M. (2016). Ambient co-presence: Transnational family practices in polymedia environments. *Global Networks, 16*(2), 183–201.

Madianou, M., & Miller, D. (2013). Polymedia: Towards a new theory of digital media in interpersonal communication. *International Journal of Cultural Studies, 16*(2), 169–187.

Malacrida, C., & Boulton, T. (2012). Women's perceptions of childbirth "choices" competing discourses of motherhood, sexuality, and selflessness. *Gender & Society, 26*(5), 748–772.

Martin, J., Sugarman, J., & Thompson, J. (2003). *Psychology and the question of agency*. Albany, NY: SUNY Press.

Mascheroni, G. Researching datafied children as data citizens. *Journal of Children and Media, 12*(4), 517–523.

Maternity Action. (2014). *Valuing families? The impact of cuts to maternity benefits since 2010*. London: Maternity Action.

McKeever, R., & McKeever, B. W. (2017). Moms and media: Exploring the effects of online communication on infant feeding practices. *Health Communication, 32*(9), 1059–1065.

McRobbie, A. (2009). *The Aftermath of Feminism: Gender, culture and social change*. London: Sage.

McRobbie, A. (2013). Feminism, the family and the new "mediated" maternalism (report). *New Formations, 80*(80–81), 119–137.

Meißner, S. (2016). Effects of quantified self beyond self-optimization. In S. Selke (ed.) *Digital self-tracking and Lifelogging – Between disruptive technology and cultural transformation* (pp. 235–248). Wiesbaden: Springer VS.

Melling, B., & Houguet-Pincham, T. (2011). Online peer support for individuals with depression: A summary of current research and future considerations. *Psychiatric Rehabilitation Journal, 34*(3), 252–254.

Miller, T. (2007). "Is this what motherhood is all about?" Weaving experiences and discourse through transition to first-time motherhood. *Gender & Society, 21*(3), 337–358.

Miller, T., Bonas, S., & Dixon-Woods, M. (2007). Qualitative research on breastfeeding in the UK: A narrative review and methodological reflection. *Evidence and Policy, 3*(2), 197–230.

Mol, A. (2000). What diagnostic devices do: The case of blood sugar measurement. *Theoretical Medicine and Bioethics, 21*(1), 9–22.

Mollen, A., & Dhaenens, F. (2018). Audiences' coping practices with intrusive interfaces: Researching audiences in algorithmic, datafied, platform societies. In R. Das & B. Ytre-Arne (eds.) *The future of audiences* (pp. 43–60). Cham: Palgrave Macmillan.

Moore, D., & Ayers, S. (2017). Virtual voices: Social support and stigma in postnatal mental illness Internet forums. *Psychology, Health & Medicine, 22*(5), 546–551.

Moravec, M. (Ed.). (2011). *Motherhood online*. Newcastle: Cambridge Scholars Publishing.

Morrison, A. (2011). "Suffused by feeling and affect": The intimate public of personal mommy blogging. *Biography, 34*(1), 37–55.

Murray, M. (2014). Back to work? Childcare negotiations and intensive mothering in Santiago de Chile. *Journal of Family Issues. 36*(9), 1171–1191.
Myrick, J. G., & Willoughby, J. F. (2017). Educated but anxious: How emotional states and education levels combine to influence online health information seeking. *Health Informatics Journal*. doi:10.1177/1460458217719561
Nadesan, M. H. (2002). Engineering the entrepreneurial infant: Brain science, infant development toys, and governmentality. *Cultural Studies, 16*(3), 401–432.
Nash, M. (2012a). Weighty matters: Negotiating "fatness" and "in-betweenness" in early pregnancy. *Feminism & Psychology, 22*(3), 307–323.
Nash, M. (2012b). *Making "postmodern" mothers: Pregnant embodiment, baby bumps and body image*. London: Springer.
National Health Service. (2016). NHS England Children's Health Digital Strategy 2016. https://www.england.nhs.uk/digitaltechnology/wp-content/uploads/sites/31/2015/12/CHIS-Digital-Strategy-2016-v6-FS-edit-with-alt-txt-2.pdf
National Health Service. (2017a). *Improving access to perinatal mental health services in England – A review*. London: NHS.
National Health Service. (2017b). Harnessing technology and innovation. Retrieved from www.england.nhs.uk/five-year-forward-view/next-steps-on-the-nhs-five-year-forward-view/harnessing-technology-and-innovation/ on 20 November 2017.
National Health Service. (2019). Digital Inclusion Guide to Health and Social Care. London: NHS.
National Information Board. (2014a). *Personalised health and care 2020*. Leeds: NHS England.
National Information Board. (2014b). *Healthy children: Transforming child health information*. Leeds: NHS England.
NCT. (2017). *The hidden half. Bringing postnatal mental illness out of hiding*. London: NCT. www.nct.org.uk/get-involved/campaigns/hidden-half-campaign
North East London Strategic Health Authority. (2003). *Report of an independent inquiry into the care & treatment of Daksha Emson & her daughter Freya*. London: NELSHA.
Nutbeam, D., McGill, B., & Premkumar, P. (2017). Improving health literacy in community populations: A review of progress. *Health Promotion International*. doi:10.1093/heapro/dax015
O'Brien Hallstein, D. L. (2011). She gives birth, she's wearing a bikini: Mobilizing the postpregnant celebrity mom body to manage the post-second wave crisis in femininity. *Women's Studies in Communication, 34*(2), 111–138.
O'Brien Hallstein and Hanson, C. (2004). *A cultural history of pregnancy: Pregnancy, medicine and culture, 1750–2000*. Berlin: Springer.
O'Connor, H., & Madge, C. (2004). "My mum's thirty years out of date" the role of the internet in the transition to motherhood. *Community Work and Family, 7*(3), 351–369. http://hdl.handle.net/2381/11456; doi:10.1080/1366880042000295754
O'Connor, T. G., Heron, J., Golding, J., Beveridge, M., & Glover, V. (2002). Maternal antenatal anxiety and children's behavioural/emotional problems at 4 years: Report from the Avon longitudinal study of parents and children. *The British Journal of Psychiatry, 180*(6), 502–508.
O'Donohoe, S., Hogg, M., Maclaran, P., Martens, L., & Stevens, L. (Eds.). (2013). *Motherhoods, markets and consumption: The making of mothers in contemporary western cultures* (Vol. 18). London: Routledge.
O'Mahony, J., & Donnelly, T. (2010). Immigrant and refugee women's postpartum depression help-seeking experiences and access to care: A review and

analysis of the literature. *Journal of Psychiatric and Mental Health Nursing, 17*(10), 917–928.

Oakley, A. (1984). *The captured womb: A history of the medical care of pregnant women.* Oxford: Blackwell.

Onozawa, K., Kumar, R. C., Adams, D., Dore, C., & Glover, V. (2003). High EPDS scores in women from ethnic minorities living in London. *Archives of Women's Mental Health, 6*(2), 51–55.

Orgad, S. (2005). The transformative potential of online communication: The case of breast cancer patients' internet spaces. *Feminist Media Studies, 5*(2), 141–161. doi:10.1080/14680770500111980

Orgad, S. (2019). *Heading home: Motherhood, work, and the failed promise of equality.* New York: Columbia University Press.

Orgad, S., & De Benedictis, S. (2015). The "stay-at-home" mother, postfeminism and neoliberalism: Content analysis of UK news coverage. *European Journal of Communication 30*(4), 418–436.

Orr, D., Baram-Tsabari, A., & Landsman, K. (2016). Social media as a platform for health-related public debates and discussions: The polio vaccine on Facebook. *Israel Journal of Health Policy Research, 5*(1), 34. doi:10.1186/s13584-016-0093-4

Orton-Johnson, K. (2017). Mummy blogs and representations of motherhood: "Bad mummies" and their readers. *Social Media+ Society, 3*(2). doi:10.1177/2056305117707186

Ouellette, L., & Wilson, J. (2011). Women's work: Affective labour and convergence culture. *Cultural Studies, 25*(4–5), 548–565.

Paasonen, S. (2011). *Carnal resonance: Affect and online pornography.* Cambridge, MA: MIT Press.

Pain, R. (2006). Paranoid parenting? Rematerializing risk and fear for children. *Social & Cultural Geography, 7*(2), 221–243.

Parker, R. (1997). The production and purposes of maternal ambivalence. In W. Hollway & B. Featherstone (eds.) *Mothering and ambivalence* (pp. 17–36). London: Routledge.

Parker, R. (2005). *Torn in two: Maternal ambivalence.* London: Virago.

Parker, R. (2009). Why study the maternal. *Studies in the Maternal,* 1(1), 1–4.

Pedersen, S. (2016). The good, the bad and the "good enough" mother on the UK parenting forum mumsnet. *Women's Studies International Forum, 59,* 32–38.

Pedersen, S., & Smithson, J. (2013, June). Mothers with attitude – How the mumsnet parenting forum offers space for new forms of femininity to emerge online. *Women's studies international forum, 38,* 97–106. Oxford: Pergamon.

Petersen, A. (1997). Risk, governance and the new public health. *Foucault, Health and Medicine.* Petersen, A. & Bunton, R., eds. London: Routledge.

Pettigrew, S., Archer, C., & Harrigan, P. (2016). A thematic analysis of mothers' motivations for blogging. *Maternal and Child Health Journal, 20*(5), 1025–1031. doi:10.1007/s10995-015-1887-7

Phoenix, A. (2019). Bringing home social hierarchies and inequalities. Paper presented at the British Sociological Association Conference, Glasgow, April 2019.

Prescott, J., & Mackie, L. (2017). "You sort of go down a rabbit hole ... You're just going to keep on searching": A qualitative study of searching online for pregnancy-related information during pregnancy. *Journal of Medical Internet Research, 19*(6), e194.

Putnam, R. D. (2000). Bowling alone: America's declining social capital. In L. Crothers & C. Lockhart (eds.) *Culture and politics* (pp. 223–234). New York: Palgrave Macmillan.

Radin, P. (2006). "To me, it's my life": Medical communication, trust, and activism in cyberspace. *Social Science & Medicine, 62*(3), 591–601.

Radway, J. (1985). *Reading the Romance.* Chapel Hill, NC: University of North Carolina Press.

Raphael-Leff, J. (2010). Healthy maternal ambivalence. *Studies in the Maternal, 2*(1), 1–15.

Riessman, C. K. (2008). *Narrative methods for the human sciences.* Los Angeles, CA; London: Sage.

Riessman, C. K. (2013). *Analysis of personal narratives. Handbook of interview research.* Jaber F Gubrium and James A. Holstein, eds. London: Sage.

Rizzo, K. M., Schiffrin, H. H., & Liss, M. (2013). Insight into the parenthood paradox: Mental health outcomes of intensive mothering. *Journal of Child and Family Studies, 22*(5), 614–620.

Rogers, M. (2015). Beyond blogging: How mothers use creative non-fiction techniques in digital environments to dislodge the mask of motherhood. *Journal of Family Studies, 21*(3), 248–260. doi:10.1080/13229400.2015.1074932

Romagnoli, A., & Wall, G. (2012). "I know I'm a good mom": Young, low-income mothers' experiences with risk perception, intensive parenting ideology and parenting education programmes. *Health, Risk & Society, 14*(3), 273–289.

Rose, N. 1999. *Powers of Freedom: Reframing political thought.* Cambridge: Cambridge University Press.

Royal College of Midwives. (2014). *Maternal Mental Health: Improving Emotional Well-Being in Post-Natal Care.* London: RCM.

Ruddick, S. (1989). *Maternal Thinking: Toward a Politics of Peace.* Boston, MA: Beacon Press.

Ruddick, S. (1994). Thinking mothers/conceiving birth. In D. Bassin, M. Honey, & M. M. Kaplan (eds.) *Representations of Motherhood* (pp. 29–45). New Haven, CT: Yale University Press.

Ryan, L. (2007). Migrant women, social networks and motherhood: The experiences of Irish nurses in Britain. *Sociology, 41*(2), 295–312.

Ryan, L. (2011). Migrants' social networks and weak ties: Accessing resources and constructing relationships post-migration. *The Sociological Review, 59*(4), 707–724.

Salih, R. (2003). *Gender in Transnationalism. Home, Longing and Belonging Among Moroccan Migrant Women.* London; New York: Routledge. (Routledge Research in Transnationalism; 11).

Sandelowski, M. (1984). *Pain, pleasure, and American childbirth: From the twilight sleep to the Read method, 1914–1960* (No. 13). London: Praeger.

Schaan, V. K., & Melzer, A. (2015). Parental mediation of children's television and video game use in Germany: Active and embedded in family processes. *Journal of Children and Media, 9*(1), 58–76. doi:10.1080/17482798.2015.997108

Silverstone, R. (1999). *Why study the media?.* London: Sage.

Silverstone, R. (2002). *Media and morality: On the rise of the mediapolis.* London: Wiley.

Slomian, J., Bruyère, O., Reginster, J. Y., & Emonts, P. (2017). The internet as a source of information used by women after childbirth to meet their need for information: A web-based survey. *Midwifery, 48*, 46–52.

Smith, M. A., & Kollock, P. (Eds.). (1999). *Communities in cyberspace*. Hove: Psychology Press.

Smith, R. (2012). Anxious mothers may disrupt babies' sleep. *The Telegraph*. Retrieved from www.telegraph.co.uk/news/health/news/9206423/Anxious-mothers-may-disrupt-babies-sleep-not-other-way-round-researchers.html on 02.08.2018

Smith-Rosenberg, C., & Rosenberg, C. (1973). The female animal: Medical and biological views of woman and her role in nineteenth-century America. *The Journal of American History, 60*(2), 332–356.

Stabile, C. A. (1992). Shooting the mother: Fetal photography and the politics of disappearance. *Camera Obscura, 10*(1), 178–205.

Stjernswärd, S., & Östman, M. (2006). Potential of e-health in relation to depression: Short survey of previous research. *Journal of Psychiatric and Mental Health Nursing, 13*(6), 698–703. doi:10.1111/j.1365-2850.2006.01017.x

Stoeber, J. & Otto, K. (2006). Positive conceptions of perfectionism: Approaches, evidence, challenges. *Personality and Social Psychology Review, 10*, 295–319.

Storr, T., Maher, J., & Swanepoel, E. (2017). Online nutrition information for pregnant women: A content analysis. *Maternal & Child Nutrition, 13*(2), e12315.

Takeshita, C. (2017). Countering technocracy: "Natural" birth in the business of being born and call the midwife. *Feminist Media Studies, 17*(3), 1–15.

The Guardian. (2016). The post-code lottery of new mothers' mental health. Retrieved from www.theguardian.com/society/2016/feb/10/mother-and-baby-units-perinatal-mental-health-service on 12.04. 2017.

The Guardian. (2018). Health visitors struggling with 'dangerously high' caseloads. Retrieved from https://www.theguardian.com/society/2018/sep/23/health-visitors-struggle-with-dangerously-high-caseloads

The Press Association. (2013). Half of English regions have cut midwifery funding. *Nursing Times*. Online access. Accessed on 19 July 2019. Retrieved from https://www.nursingtimes.net/archive/half-of-english-regions-have-cut-midwifery-funding-14-11-2013/

Theodorou, E., & Spyrou, S. (2013). Motherhood in utero: Consuming away anxiety. *Journal of Consumer Culture, 13*(2), 79–96.

Thompson, J. B. (1995). *The Media and Modernity: A Social Theory of the Media*. Stanford, CA: Stanford University Press.

Tulloch, J., & Lupton, D. (2003). *Risk and Everyday Life*. London: Sage.

Tyler, I. (2000). 17 reframing pregnant embodiment. In S. Ahmed et al. (eds.) *Transformations: thinking through feminism* (pp. 288–302). London: Routledge.

Tyler, I. (2009). Introduction: Birth. *Feminist Review, 93*, 1–7.

Tyler, I. (2011). Pregnant beauty: Maternal femininities under neoliberalism. In R. Gill & C. Schaffer (eds.) *New Femininities: Postfeminism, Neoliberalism and Subjectivity* (pp. 21–36). London: Palgrave Macmillan.

Tyler, I. (2013). *Revolting Subjects: Social Abjection and Resistance in Neoliberal Britain*. London: Zed Books.

Tyler, I., & Baraitser, L. (2013). Private view, public birth: Making feminist sense of the new visual culture of childbirth. *Studies in the Maternal, 5*(2), 1–27.

UN (United Nations). (2015). United Nations millennium development goals.

Valkenburg, P. M. & Peter, J. (2011). Online communication among adolescents: An integrated model of its attraction, opportunities, and risks. *Journal of Adolescent Health, 48*(2), 121–127.

Valkenburg, P. M., & Peter, J. (2007). Online communication and adolescent well-being: Testing the stimulation versus the displacement hypothesis. *Journal of Computer-Mediated Communication, 12*(4), 1169–1182.

Valkenburg, P. M., Peter, J., & Schouten, A. P. (2006). Friend networking sites and their relationship to adolescents' well-being and social self-esteem. *CyberPsychology & Behavior, 9*(5), 584–590.

Van den Bergh, B. R., & Marcoen, A. (2004). High antenatal maternal anxiety is related to ADHD symptoms, externalizing problems, and anxiety in 8-and 9-year-olds. *Child Development, 75*(4), 1085–1097.

Van den Bergh, B. R., Mulder, E. J., Mennes, M., & Glover, V. (2005). Antenatal maternal anxiety and stress and the neurobehavioural development of the fetus and child: Links and possible mechanisms. A review. *Neuroscience & Biobehavioral Reviews, 29*(2), 237–258.

Van Dijck, J. (2013). 'You have one identity': performing the self on Facebook and LinkedIn. *Media, Culture and Society, 35*(2), 199–215.

Van Dijck, J. (2014). Datafication, dataism and dataveillance: Big Data between scientific paradigm and ideology. *Surveillance & Society, 12*(2), 197–208.

Van Leeuwen, T., & Jewitt, C. (2001). *The Handbook of Visual Analysis.* London: Sage.

Vesnić-Alujević, L. Stehling, A., Jorge, A., and Marôpo, L. (2018). The co-option of audience data and user-generated content: Empowerment and exploitation amidst algorithms, produsage and crowdsourcing. In R. Das, B. Ytre-Arne (eds.) *The future of audiences* (pp. 79–99). Cham: Palgrave Macmillan.

Vivienne, S., & Burgess, J. (2012). The digital storyteller's stage: Queer everyday activists negotiating privacy and publicness. *Journal of Broadcasting & Electronic Media, 56*(3), 362–377.

Vivienne, S. & Burgess, J. (2013). The remediation of the personal photograph and the politics of self-representation in digital storytelling. *Journal of Material Culture, 18*(3), 279–298.

Wall, G. (2001). Moral constructions of motherhood in breastfeeding discourse. *Gender & Society, 15*(4), 592–610.

Wall, G. (2010). 'Mothers' experiences with intensive parenting and brain development discourse', *Women's Studies International Forum, 33*(3), 253–263.

Warner, D., & Procaccino, J. D. (2004). Toward wellness: Women seeking health information. *Journal of the Association for Information Science and Technology, 55*(8), 709–730.

Wellman, B., & Gulia, M. (1999). Net surfers don't ride alone: Virtual communities as communities. In B. Wellman (ed.) *Networks in the global village* (pp. 331–366). Boulder, CO: Westview Press.

Wellman, B., Salaff, J., Dimitrova, D., Garton, L., Gulia, M., & Haythornthwaite, C. (1996). Computer networks as social networks: Collaborative work, telework, and virtual community. *Annual Review of Sociology, 22*(1), 213–238.

White, M., & Dorman, S. M. (2001). Receiving social support online: Implications for health education. *Health Education Research, 16*(6), 693–707.

Whiteman, N. (2012). *Undoing ethics: Rethinking practice in online research.* Boston, MA: Springer US. doi:10.1007/978-1-4614-1827-6

Williams, K., Donaghue, N., & Kurz, T. (2013). "Giving guilt the flick"? An investigation of mothers' talk about guilt in relation to infant feeding. *Psychology of Women Quarterly, 37*(1), 97–112.

Wilson, J. A., & Yochim, E. C. (2015). Mothering through precarity: Becoming mamapreneurial. *Cultural Studies, 29*(5–6), 669–686.

Winderman, E. (2016). Times for birth: Chronic and kairotic mediated temporalities in TLC's a baby story. *Feminist Media Studies, 17*(3), 1–15.

Wolf, J. B. (2011). *Is Breast Best?: Taking on the Breastfeeding Experts and the New High Stakes of Motherhood.* New York: New York University Press.

Woolgar, S. (Ed.). (2002). *Virtual Society?: Technology, Cyberbole, Reality.* Oxford: Oxford University Press.

World Health Organization. (1992). *International Statistical Classification of Diseases and Related Health Problems.* 2. Geneva: World Health Organization. 30–88.

Yadlon, S. (1997). Skinny women and good mothers: The rhetoric of risk, control, and culpability in the production of knowledge about breast cancer. *Feminist Studies, 23*(3), 645–677.

Yeshua-Katz, D., & Hard, Y. (2019). Locked out of online social support: Boundary work in stigmatized communities. Paper presented at the International Communication Association Conference, Washington, DC, May 2019.

Zoonen, L. V. (2001). Feminist internet studies. *Feminist Media Studies, 1*(1), 67–72. doi:10.1080/14680770120042864

Index